Recurrent Pregnancy Loss and Adverse Natal Outcomes

Recurrent Pregnancy Loss and Adverse Natal Outcomes

Edited by
Minakshi Rohilla

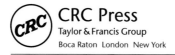

CRC Press
Taylor & Francis Group
Boca Raton London New York

CRC Press is an imprint of the
Taylor & Francis Group, an **informa** business

CRC Press
Taylor & Francis Group
6000 Broken Sound Parkway NW, Suite 300
Boca Raton, FL 33487-2742

First issued in paperback 2021

ISBN-13: 978-1-138-35182-0 (hbk)
ISBN-13: 978-1-03-217348-1 (pbk)
DOI: 10.1201/9780429435027

This book contains information obtained from authentic and highly regarded sources. Reasonable efforts have been made to publish reliable data and information, but the author and publisher cannot assume responsibility for the validity of all materials or the consequences of their use. The authors and publishers have attempted to trace the copyright holders of all material reproduced in this publication and apologize to copyright holders if permission to publish in this form has not been obtained. If any copyright material has not been acknowledged please write and let us know so we may rectify in any future reprint.

Publisher's Note

The publisher has gone to great lengths to ensure the quality of this reprint but points out that some imperfections in the original copies may be apparent.

Library of Congress Cataloging-in-Publication Data
Names: Rohilla, Minakshi, editor.
Title: Recurrent pregnancy loss and adverse natal outcomes / edited by
    Minakshi Rohilla.
Description: Boca Raton : CRC Press, 2020. | Includes bibliographical
    references and index. | Summary: "Recurrent Pregnancy Loss (RPL)
    includes recurrent first, second trimester abortions and recurrent
    preterm delivery, second or third trimester intrauterine fetal death,
    intrapartum stillbirth and early neonatal death. This book includes
    protocols for case scenarios of early and late pregnancy loss and covers
    instances of poor obstetric history"-- Provided by publisher.
Identifiers: LCCN 2020002771 (print) | LCCN 2020002772 (ebook) | ISBN
    9781138351820 (hardback) | ISBN 9780429435027 (ebook)
Subjects: MESH: Abortion, Habitual | Pregnancy Complications
Classification: LCC RG571 (print) | LCC RG571 (ebook) | NLM WQ 225 | DDC
    618.3--dc23
LC record available at https://lccn.loc.gov/2020002771
LC ebook record available at https://lccn.loc.gov/2020002772

Visit the Taylor & Francis Web site at
http://www.taylorandfrancis.com

and the CRC Press Web site at
http://www.crcpress.com

This book is dedicated to my father, the late Sh. Ram Kishore Rohilla, and my mother Smt. Luxmi Devi Rohilla.

Contents

Preface

High-risk pregnancy with a history of recurrent pregnancy loss and previous adverse pregnancy outcome is a challenging condition not uncommonly faced by an obstetrician in day-to-day practice. Recurrent pregnancy loss is a multifactorial entity with variable etiology and even more variable management options. Besides obstetrics, the management of recurrent pregnancy loss often requires an intricate interaction between different related disciplines such as neonatology, genetics, internal medicine, endocrinology, and immunology. It is essential that every consultant and trainee have a thorough and dedicated knowledge about investigations, management, and approaches to these women.

Management of recurrent pregnancy loss has always been a dilemma for the affected couple and treating obstetrician. Although many advances have been made in the last few years in understanding and managing recurrent pregnancy loss, its unexplained cause frequently eludes us. It has been my passion to develop a practical approach for the management of pregnancy with a history of recurrent pregnancy loss for those involved in managing these women. Unrelenting effort has gone into this book in order to present an approach to these pregnancies, from first- and second-trimester pregnancy loss to stillbirths and late neonatal deaths. Management of women with a previous child with intellectual disability or a syndromic child has also been added for the sake of completeness of the subject.

The hope is that this book will be a handy reference for those interested in this subject matter and will serve as easy reading for consultant gynecologists, trainees, and especially all those working in the field of high-risk pregnancy and adverse pregnancy outcomes. Each chapter ends with a summary of the covered approach to women with recurrent pregnancy loss, and the concerned subject has been highlighted with figures and flowcharts. The journey to completion of this book has been a learning, informative, and satisfying experience, and the wish is for the reader to share in that experience.

Minakshi Rohilla, MD

Acknowledgments

I gratefully acknowledge the efforts of my fellow colleagues who despite their busy schedules of patient care worked diligently to contribute the various chapters. Their help in completion and editing was appreciated. I would like to thank my family for their constant encouragement in timely completion of this book. I would also like to express gratitude to my teachers who painstakingly taught me this subject and made me capable of taking up the arduous task of writing this book. My sincere thanks are due to all the patients of this subject, who proved to be the ultimate teachers to my learning.

Editor

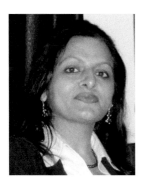

Minakshi Rohilla, MD, is professor of obstetrics and gynecology at the Department of Obstetrics and Gynecology at the Postgraduate Institute of Medical Education and Research (PGIMER), Chandigarh (U.T), India.

She served as consultant in charge of the Recurrent Pregnancy Loss (RPL) clinic since 2008 and was appointed as core faculty for a fellowship in high-risk pregnancy and perinatology. She has published more than 55 papers in reputed journals and has served as a faculty member since 2005 in this premier service organization of India.

She obtained her medical science (MBBS) degree from Allahabad University (U.P), India, and her MD from the University of Lucknow (U.P), India. She has guided several students in completing their master's degree dissertations on different causes of recurrent pregnancy loss, such as immunologic aspects, inherited thrombophilia, previous stillbirths, and thyroid autoimmunity with obstetric outcomes in women with recurrent miscarriage.

Contributors

KG Amulya
PGIMER
Chandigarh, India

Ashima Arora
PGIMER
Chandigarh, India

Richa Arora
PGIMER
Chandigarh, India

Darshan Hosapatna Basavarajappa
PGIMER
Chandigarh, India

Seema Chopra
PGIMER
Chandigarh, India

Shalini Gainder
PGIMER
Chandigarh, India

Surbhi Gupta
PGIMER
Chandigarh, India

Bharti Joshi
PGIMER
Chandigarh, India

Deepmala Modi
PGIMER
Chandigarh, India

Tanuja Muthyala
AIIMS Mangalgiri
Andhra Pradesh, India

Minakshi Rohilla
PGIMER
Chandigarh, India

Pradip Kumar Saha
PGIMER
Chandigarh, India

Bharti Sharma
PGIMER
Chandigarh, India

Shivani Sharma
PGIMER
Chandigarh, India

Pooja Sikka
PGIMER
Chandigarh, India

Aruna Singh
PGIMER
Chandigarh, India

Rimpi Singla
PGIMER
Chandigarh, India

Sujata Siwatch
PGIMER
Chandigarh, India

Approach to women with recurrent first-trimester abortions: Need of the hour

TANUJA MUTHYALA

PROBLEM BURDEN

Around 5% of women of reproductive age experience two consecutive miscarriages, and less than 1% experience three or more miscarriages consecutively [1]. There is a scarcity of data on exact prevalence of recurrent pregnancy loss (RPL) in the first trimester, and the exact numbers cannot be determined because not all pregnancies are reported; some abort unnoticed, some are biochemical pregnancies, and the rest are lost due to recall or reporting bias. The prevalence of RPL varies widely due to diverse demographic profiles and lack of a universal or standardized definition to categorize RPL.

The incidence of sporadic pregnancy loss is around 25%–30%, and 1%–2% experience RPL as per data from epidemiological studies [2]. The incidence is relatively higher in older and infertile couples. The numbers are on the rise due to late marriages, advanced maternal age, and lifestyle modifications. In Sweden, the incidence of RPL increased by 74% over a 10-year study period, 2003–2012 [3].

ECONOMIC BURDEN

Costs incurred for managing patients with RPL involve managing index pregnancy and workup for RPL. If the current pregnancy loss does not abort spontaneously, medical or surgical curettage is required. The cost for evidence-based workup for RPL is estimated at $3551, and if extensive workup is required, including screen for thrombophilia, it sums up to $5176. The cost estimate for karyotyping of products of conception (POCs) is $1128 and for office-based manual vacuum aspiration is $1338. In order to lower these costs, Nastaran et al. [4] compared the cost-effectiveness of getting a karyotype of POC in the second loss as an initial step. If POCs are euploid or have inconclusive karyotype results, then the couple should proceed for further workup. If the karyotype results are suggestive of an aneuploid fetus, the couple would

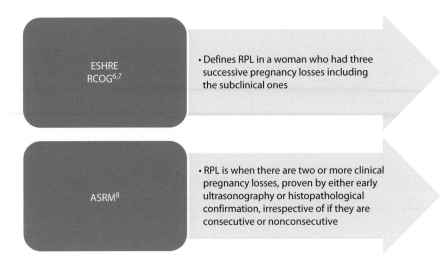

Figure 1.1 Definition of recurrent pregnancy loss.

not proceed for further evaluation. Thus, it is more cost effective and saves $1135 for that particular age group. Cost estimates may be more accurate if hospital visits and sessions for psychological counseling are added, as these couples are more prone to depression and other behavioral changes [4].

DEFINITION OF RECURRENT PREGNANCY LOSS

The World Health Organization defines miscarriage as loss of pregnancy before attaining viability [5]. Various terminologies used for RPL are *recurrent miscarriage* or *habitual abortion*. Different definitions and classifications have been used by different societies [6–9] (Figures 1.1 and 1.2).

RISK FACTORS FOR RPL

Probable risk for subsequent pregnancy to abort after two successive losses is around 25% and after three losses is around 30%. Therefore, it is prudent to initiate workup for RPL after two losses and earlier if the couple is infertile or female age is older than 35 years [10].

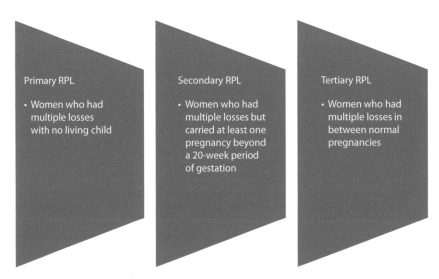

Figure 1.2 Classification of recurrent pregnancy loss. (From Silver RM et al., *Obstet Gynecol.* 2011;118[6]:1402–8.)

MODIFIABLE AND NONMODIFIABLE RISK FACTORS

Nonmodifiable risk factors

1. *Age*: Prognostication of a couple with RPL is done on the basis of female age and the number of prior pregnancy losses. Pregnancies with advanced-age couples—women 35 years or older and men 40 years or older—tend to have unfavorable outcomes as compared to women of 20–35 years of age. The line diagram presented in Figure 1.3 suggests that with increasing maternal age, the risk for early pregnancy loss increases [11,12].

2. *Obstetric history*: Obstetric history predicts subsequent pregnancy outcomes. With every abortion, a woman's risk of subsequent loss increases and is approximately 40% after three consecutive pregnancy losses. History of live birth does not necessarily decrease the risk of future loss. However, even after four consecutive losses, the probability of the next pregnancy reaching term is 60%–65% [13]. There are studies reporting an unfavorable course of events in subsequent pregnancies both antepartum and intrapartum in women with RPL. Reported are obstetric complications such as threatened abortion, hypertensive disorders of pregnancy, malpresentations, antepartum and postpartum hemorrhage, induction of labor, instrumental deliveries, and manual removal of placenta. Thus, women with primary RPLs behave like "virtual primigravidae" in their subsequent pregnancy and experience labor characteristics, complications, and perinatal outcomes similar to primigravidae [13,14]. In a review study, Hammoud et al. noticed that the risk of preterm delivery is directly proportional to the number of miscarriages; perinatal mortality was high because of preterm births in women with primary RPL. The association between these two is difficult to explain as early pregnancy loss is secondary to implantation defect, and preterm labor occurs later in gestation. The possible explanation for this may be secondary to repeated dilatation and curettages indicated in previous early losses [15].

3. *Gestational age at loss*: Etiology for abortions in the first trimester differs from those that occur in the second trimester and thus outcomes vary. Loss after documented report of obtaining fetal cardiac activity has a poorer prognosis than that of a loss of a nonviable gestation [13].

Modifiable risk factors

LIFESTYLE AND ENVIRONMENTAL FACTORS

1. *Body mass index*: Raised BMI is independently associated with higher miscarriage rates. Obese women who become pregnant after successful fertility treatment are more likely to experience miscarriage than those who conceive spontaneously. The results of genetic analysis of products of conception from 204 abortions when correlated with maternal age and BMI are shown in Table 1.1 [16].

   Semen parameters and unexplained RPL: A cross-sectional study of 305 men attending urology clinic compared semen analysis and DNA fragmentation assays of overweight (BMI $\geq$ 25 kg/m^2 <30) and obese ($\geq$30 kg/m^2) with normal weight men (<25 kg/m^2) and interpreted that the percentage of DNA damage was significantly higher in obese men [17]. Sperm

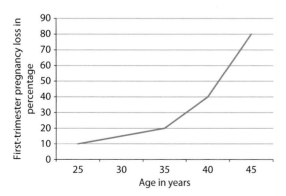

Figure 1.3 Relation between maternal age and probability of early pregnancy loss in percentage.

Table 1.1 Comparison of maternal age and body mass index (BMI) to euploid and aneuploid fetuses

Risk factor		Euploid fetus	Aneuploid fetus	P value
Age (years)	<35	51%	40%	0.009
	>35	32%	68%	
BMI (kg/m^2)	<25	37%	63%	0.040
	$\geq$25	53%	47%	

from couples with a history of RPL showed an increase in sex chromosomal disomy. A study by Carrell reported a significantly increased mean aneuploidy rate in couples with unexplained RPL compared with the control groups [18].

2. *Alcohol, smoking or tobacco chewing, caffeine intake in women*: When a one-to-one comparison is done, each of these has a weaker association as compared to sporadic loss when taken in usual doses. However, fertilization rates are negatively affected in men who smoke and are alcoholics.

3. *Occupational exposure to radiation/heavy metals/pollutants*: There is no significant increased risk, when individually compared. However, the risk score of RPL increases when men who are occupationally exposed also have other risk factors such as smoking and alcohol consumption. De Fleurian et al. [19] observed abnormal semen parameters in men with exposure to heavy metals, solvent fumes, and polycyclic aromatic hydrocarbons, and reciprocally in those who had abnormal semen analysis reports, the mean exposure index to pesticides and other chemicals was significantly higher when compared to those with normal semen analysis [20]. Table 1.2 depicts the relationship of modifiable risk factors with RPL.

Approach to women with recurrent first-trimester abortions

Recurrence suggests a persistent cause that must be identified and treated. This is not always true, as even with extensive workup, cause is ascertained in only 60% of couples. Screening and treating the cause, thorough counseling, and explaining possible future risks, recurrence rates, and regular follow-up of these patients in clinics dedicated to RPL has a better pregnancy outcome [2]. Workup can be classified into evidence-based and extensive workup. Figure 1.4 demonstrates the approach to women with RPL in the first trimester.

Table 1.2 Modifiable risk factors and their relationship with recurrent pregnancy loss

Risk factor	Evidence	Study	Inference
BMI	Rittenberg et al. [21], Boots et al. [22]	Retrospective study of 393 women undergoing IVF	Risk of miscarriage is two times higher in women with BMI >25 kg/m^2 compared to BMI of 18.5–24.9. If BMI >30 kg/m^2, risk of spontaneous loss is 27% higher. In women with RPL and BMI >30 kg/m^2, probability of spontaneous miscarriage was 7% higher.
Alcohol	Rasch [23]	Case control study	Increased risk with more than three drinks per week in the first trimester (OR 2.3) or more than five drinks per week throughout pregnancy.
Caffeine	Cnattingius et al. [24]	Case control study	Risk of loss increases with intake of three to five cups of coffee per day, and the higher the uptake, the higher the risk of abortion.
Stress	Plana-Ripoll et al. [25]	Cohort study	Stress and RPL are interlinked; however, whether it is the cause or effect is not clear.
Smoking	ESHRE guidelines [6]	Evidence-based recommendations	Smoking affects sperm quality, implantation rates, endometrial receptivity, and live birth rates; therefore, couples with RPL should be counseled against smoking.

Abbreviations: BMI, body mass index; ESHRE, European Society of Human Reproduction and Embryology; IVF, *in vitro* fertilization; OR, odds ratio; RPL, recurrent pregnancy loss.

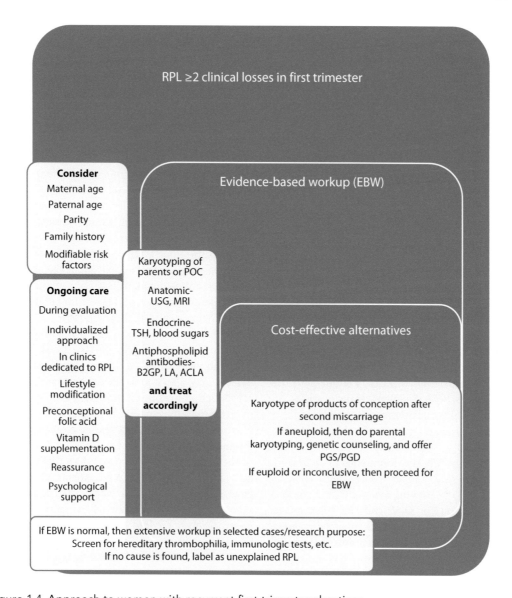

Figure 1.4 Approach to women with recurrent first-trimester abortions.

Evidence-based workup

Evidence-based workup includes genetic evaluation of the couple, evaluation for anatomical and endocrine factors, and testing for antiphospholipid antibodies. The literature suggests that identifying and treating these causes may lead to a favorable outcome in successive pregnancies. As subfertile couples have relatively higher rates of spontaneous abortions, and more than one cause may prevail, these couples require early evaluation, as early as even after a single loss. Embryonic losses or recurrent first-trimester abortions occur more commonly following chromosomal aberrations, and others may be secondary to antiphospholipid antibodies, endocrine factors, inherited thrombophilias (deficiency of antithrombin-III, protein C, or protein S; mutations in factor V Leiden or prothrombin gene; and hyperhomocysteinemia), and rarely anatomical or infectious causes.

Genetic causes

The most common cause of first-trimester abortion is genetic, which includes chromosomal aberrations that are embryonic or parental in origin. These are

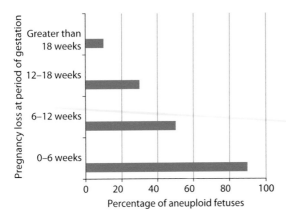

Figure 1.5 Comparison of gestational age in weeks at pregnancy loss to percentage of aneuploidy.

seen in around 75% of pregnancy tissue specimens following spontaneous first-trimester abortions. It may be a balanced (2%–5% of couples) or unbalanced translocation, embryonic aneuploidy, numerical error (most commonly a trisomy), gene duplication or deletion, or rarely a single-gene disorder. Couples with balanced translocations are less likely to deliver a live-born affected child [2].

With every abortion, risk of subsequent pregnancy loss due to a genetic factor decreases; thus, in women with RPL, the occurrence of embryonic aneuploidy is less than in women with sporadic miscarriages [7]. Carrying a fetus with an unbalanced translocation may end in miscarriage/stillbirth or as a live birth with major congenital malformations. When pregnancy losses from different periods of gestation were compared, the probability of loss due to aneuploidy decreased with advancing gestation as shown in Figure 1.5 [26]. The American College of Obstetricians and Gynecologists (ACOG) recommends genetic analysis of products of conception for women who had two successive or three nonsuccessive abortions [2].

Genetic analysis

At present, genetic testing is used for diagnosis and for prognosticating.

PRODUCTS OF CONCEPTION

Products of conception are subjected to an array-based comparative genomic hybridization (array-CGH) to reduce maternal contamination [27]. A thorough and cost-effective approach by selective evaluation for RPL is done. Selective evaluation implies further evaluation should be done only if the karyotyping results are suggestive of a euploid fetus. This cost-effective approach holds true even for advanced maternal age. On the contrary, universal evaluation indicates a panel of investigations for every couple after a second miscarriage [28].

PARENTAL GENETIC TESTING

Peripheral blood karyotyping may reveal numeric and structural cytogenetic abnormalities, which are the most thoroughly investigated genetic causes of RPL. Both the specific chromosome(s) affected and type of rearrangement influence the probability of a future live birth. Genetic counseling gives an idea to the affected couple about the chances of transmission of the identified abnormality, risk of future pregnancy loss, and possibility of delivering a live affected child if they choose to continue to attempt pregnancy spontaneously without intervention. Known carriers of structural chromosome abnormalities and some with single-gene defects may also choose to proceed with assisted reproduction in combination with genetic analysis of resulting embryos via preimplantation genetic diagnosis (PGD) to select against embryo transfer. Parental karyotype abnormalities are transmitted to the fetus at a frequency less than that predicted by Mendelian genetics. In a cohort study by Carp et al., known parental karyotype aberrations were seen in only 10% of abortus, whereas 43.5% of abortuses were euploid [29]. This variation may be due to preclinical loss of some affected embryos. In the case of abnormal parental karyotype, the couple can still be encouraged to conceive naturally, as aberrations in parental karyotyping might not be directly predictive of subsequent embryonic karyotype abnormalities. There is a 75% chance of delivering a healthy baby versus possible risk of recurrence of 5%–10%, which may result in spontaneous miscarriage again or if continued may need to use prenatal diagnostic techniques like chorionic villous sampling in the first trimester for genetic assay. Couples who do not opt for this can be advised about gamete donation or adoption [30].

However, there are no recommendations supporting use or favorable outcomes with their use, even with the recently advanced PGS methods. In 2008, the American Society for Reproductive Medicine (ASRM), the European Society of Human Reproduction and Embryology (ESHRE), and the British Fertility Society were of the opinion that when PGS was routinely offered, there was no significant improvement in pregnancy outcomes. Availing PGS had no increased perinatal outcomes; on the contrary, it was costly and invasive. Rather a conservative and teamwork-based approach focusing on supportive care with regular monitoring is advised [31].

SINGLE-GENE DEFECTS

Single-gene defects associated with pregnancy loss include musculoskeletal gene mutations including trinucleotide repeat sequences, genes involved in immune system regulation, pregnancy implantation, thrombophilic gene mutations, and mutations in specific enzymes. These causes for recurrent first-trimester loss are rare.

Endocrinal/hormonal screen

Uncontrolled diabetes mellitus, thyroid disorders, and symptomatic hyperprolactinemia should be investigated and treated. Treatment options or supportive treatment in RPL with polycystic ovarian syndrome and luteal phase defects are similar to women without RPL.

DIABETES MELLITUS AND RPL

Pregnancy losses are increased at the extremes of glycemia in both normal and diabetic pregnancy but at higher levels in diabetic pregnancy. Pregestational diabetes is clearly associated with increased risk, but it is unclear whether subclinical glucose intolerance is associated with RPL [32]. The American Diabetes Association suggests the following glycemic targets for women with preexisting diabetes anxious to conceive: fasting sugar of 60–99 mg/dL, postprandial sugars of 100–129 mg/dL, with HbA1C less than 6% [33]. Diabetic women who had a spontaneous abortion had higher fasting and postprandial glucose levels than those delivering a live infant at term. Risk of pregnancy loss was higher with higher HbA1C levels. For example, one standard deviation increase in first-trimester HbA1C from normal had a 3.1% increase in the rate of pregnancy loss, and a four standard deviation increase had a 40% pregnancy loss rate [34].

Women on SGLT1 (sodium glucose transporter 1) inhibitors like sotagliflozin for treatment of diabetes should be advised against their use in pregnancy. SGLT1 is expressed in the endometrium and controls glycogen accumulation essential for histiotrophic nutrition in pregnancy. Relative SGLT1 deficiency in the human endometrium at implantation may predispose for early pregnancy failure and obstetric complications, including fetal growth restriction [35].

THYROID DISORDERS AND RPL

Screening for thyroid disorders is done by estimating serum concentrations of thyrotropin (TSH), thyroid peroxidase antibodies (anti-TPO) and T4 (thyroxin) levels if either of them is abnormal [36].

SERUM THYROTROPIN VALUES IN PREGNANCY

The 2017 American Thyroid Association guidelines in pregnancy recommend that an upper reference limit of 4.0 mU/L can be used if local population reference normal values are not available. However, TSH of 4.0 mU/L is high, and many cases of subclinical hypothyroidism may be missed; therefore, a value of 3.0 mU/L in the first trimester and 3.5 in the second and third trimesters can be considered until nationally representative data for trimester-specific TSH values are generated [37,38].

THYROID PEROXIDASE ANTIBODIES AND RPL

The association between RPL and raised levels of TPO antibodies is controversial. In a large cohort study with 5914 women with RPL, the presence of TPO antibodies did not increase the incidence of euploid miscarriage or adverse pregnancy outcome. In the TABLET trial, the use of levothyroxine in those with elevated anti-TPO levels *did not* decrease the risk of abortion in trial participants and it did not result in a higher rate of live births beyond 34 weeks [39]. However, if RPL is caused by an immunologic reaction, thyroid autoimmunity does not seem to be a sensitive marker. A meta-analysis of eight studies that included 460 Ab-positive patients and 1923 controls noted a significant association between thyroid Ab positivity and recurrent pregnancy loss (odds ratio [OR] 2.3, 95% confidence interval [CI] 1.5–3.5) [40,41]. Kim and colleagues reported that women with recurrent pregnancy loss who were antithyroid Ab-positive also demonstrated higher levels of anticardiolipin Ab and other non-organ-specific antibodies [42].

Insufficient evidence exists to conclusively determine whether LT4 therapy decreases pregnancy loss risk in TPOAb-positive euthyroid women who are newly pregnant. However, administration of LT4 to TPOAb-positive euthyroid pregnant women with a prior history of loss may be considered given its potential benefits in comparison with its minimal risk. In such cases, 25–50 μg of LT4 is a typical starting dose [43].

In a case control study by Lata et al., the prevalence of thyroid autoimmunity was much higher (31%) in pregnant women with a history of RPL than in the healthy pregnant control population. After treatment with LT4 therapy there was no difference in prevalence of miscarriage between euthyroid and hypothyroid TPOAb-positive women [44].

POLYCYSTIC OVARY SYNDROME AND RPL

RPL in PCOS occurs in around half of total pregnancies [45]. However, the treatment for women with PCOS with or without RPL remains the same. The postulated mechanisms in PCOS linked to RPL are as follows [45]:

1. Hyperandrogenemia, hyperinsulinemia, and increased insulin resistance (IR) found in PCOS patients are also individually associated with increased risk of miscarriage. Wang et al. noticed higher IR in early trimesters in women with a history of RPL.
2. PCOS involves several confounding factors that may contribute, individually or in combination, to thrombosis and eventually lead to RPL [45].
3. Among all hypotheses, IR, obesity, and hyperhomocysteinemia (HHcy) play significant roles in RPL. The incidence of HHcy and IR was 70% and 56%, respectively, in the RPL-affected PCOS population, which was significantly higher as compared to the non-PCOS group (HHcy: 57%; IR: 6%). Rates of miscarriage were significantly greater in HHcy-induced miscarriage when compared to the normohomocysteinemic segment (PCOS: 70% versus 29% and non-PCOS: 57% versus 42%) along with the IR population (PCOS: 70% versus 56% and non-PCOS: 57% versus 6%) in both groups [46].
4. Raised PAI-I (an endogenous inhibitor of fibrinolysis) levels with hypofibrinolysis resulting in thrombosis have an independent association with RPL in women in this polycystic ovarian syndrome (PCOS) [46].
5. Celik et al. compared 64 pregnant women with RPL to 64 pregnant controls and found

significantly higher mean values of fasting blood glucose, fasting serum insulin, and HOMA-IR (homeostatic model assessment of insulin resistance) in the RPL group [47]. Jakubowicz et al. found that hyperinsulinemia led to reduced concentrations of insulin-like growth factor binding protein-1 (IGFBP-1) and glycodelin in the early stage of pregnancy, thereby increasing the likelihood for miscarriage. Glycodelin may play a role in inhibiting the endometrial immune response of the embryo, and IGFBP-1 appears to facilitate adhesion processes at the fetal-maternal interface. Insulin, however, can negatively regulate the concentrations of glycodelin and IGFBP-1, increasing the risk for miscarriage [48].

HYPERPROLACTINEMIA AND RPL

High serum prolactin levels cause impaired folliculogenesis, oocyte dysmaturation, and a shortened luteal phase. When such women were treated with bromocriptine in subsequent pregnancy, the treated group had an 85% live birth rate and the control group had a 52% live birth rate [49].

FERTILITY HORMONES AND RPL

Interferon (IFN)-γ was found to be an emerging factor responsible in the etiology of miscarriage in association with luteinizing hormone (LH) and prolactin. The serum levels of prolactin, follicle-stimulating hormone (FSH), and LH increased significantly in the RPL group compared to the control. The hypersecretion of LH tends to be strongly associated with subfertility and early pregnancy failure [49].

AUTOIMMUNITY AND RPL

Approximately 20% of women with RPL have autoimmune etiologies, and antiphospholipid antibody (aPL) syndrome is one of the most common autoimmune etiologic factors for RPL. Approximately 15% of women with three or more RPLs have persistently positive aPL, and the fetal loss rate is around 50%–90% if no treatment was given. It is the most commonly diagnosed and treatable entity and is the only proven thrombophilia with documented adverse pregnancy outcome. The obstetric diagnostic criteria are three or more embryonic losses, one or more fetal loss of more than 10 weeks' gestation, history of preeclampsia leading to fetal growth restriction and premature birth, raised titers of lupus anticoagulant, β2-glycoprotein, or anticardiolipin antibodies. Mechanisms contributing to RPL include the following:

1. *Inflammation*: It is the core of the pathogenesis of this syndrome, and tissue injury is the result of complement-mediated inflammatory reaction in addition to thrombosis.
2. *Endometrial and subendometrial vascularity*: Measured by Doppler ultrasound, these vascularities were significantly impaired in women with RPL and aPL during the midluteal phase compared with normal fertile women, thus affecting implantation rates.

These women should be started on low-dose aspirin preconception and anticoagulation when urine pregnancy test is positive and continued for at least 6 weeks postpartum. Aspirin and antithrombotics can also stimulate IL-3, an essential factor for implantation and placental growth; hence, more favorable embryonic implantation may be induced. In a recent meta-analysis by Ziakas, heparin treatment was reported to be effective in early pregnancy loss in aPL patients but not in late pregnancy loss. When low molecular weight heparin (LMWH) and aspirin treatment was directly compared with unfractionated heparin (UFH) and aspirin treatment, there were no differences in pregnancy outcome [50,51]. D'Ippolito et al. proved that LMWH is able to antagonize the detrimental effects of aPL on human endometrial endothelial cells by disrupting the interaction of b2GPI with aPLs on the surface of these cells in a dose-dependent manner [52]. Though statistics suggest improvement in live birth rates following treatment, the effect on other obstetric variables like fetal growth restriction and preeclampsia is not satisfactory enough. There is no added benefit of corticosteroids in women with RPL secondary to anti phospholipid antibody (APLA), who are receiving aspirin and heparin. Other autoimmune disorders like systemic lupus erythematous, inflammatory bowel disease, autoimmune thyroiditis, celiac disease, and even high titer autoantibodies not fitting into any syndrome were found to be associated with RPL [53].

Anatomical cause

Cervical incompetence and congenital uterine anomalies such as a septate, bicornuate uterus usually lead to midtrimester loss. In septate uterus, if the implantation occurs on the septum which is a less vascularized fibromuscular tissue, it hinders effective fetal vascularization or placental development and thus may cause first-trimester abortion. Septal resection under hysterolaparoscopic guidance decreased abortion rates from 80% to 20% and a successful pregnancy outcome from 20% to 90% in one study [2]. Transabdominal and transvaginal three- or four-dimensional ultrasound is recommended to identify uterine anomalies [2].

Extensive workup

THROMBOPHILIA SCREEN

Inherited thrombophilias cause thrombosis of uteroplacental vasculature, which may result in recurrent abortions or more commonly stillbirth or fetal growth restriction (Table 1.3).

ACOG does not routinely recommend screening for hereditary thrombophilias, and the Royal College of Obstetricians and Gynaecologists (RCOG) does not suggest empirical treatment with anticoagulants unless medically indicated [2,54]. Viser et al. reported similar birth rates in women with RPL and hereditary thrombophilias when treated with either aspirin or heparin or both. Hyperhomocystinemia has prothrombotic potential and can cause vascular thrombosis and may lead to abortions. Screen for serum homocysteine levels can be done in unexplained cases of RPL. Treatment is by supplemental folic acid, and uncontrolled or severe hyperhomocystinemias may require prophylactic anticoagulation [54,55].

Table 1.3 Hereditary thrombophilias associated with recurrent pregnancy loss

Hereditary thrombophilias associated with RPL

Factor V Leiden mutation: In deficient or carrier status, doubles the risk of RPL

Prothrombin G20210A mutation: In deficient or carrier status, doubles the risk of RPL

Antithrombin III deficiency

Protein C deficiency

Protein S deficiency

Hyperhomocysteinemia due to mutations of methylenetetrahydrofolate reductase (*MTHFR*) gene

In a study from Northern part of India Kumar et al. investigated inherited thrombophilia in women with recurrent miscarriages, heterozygous FVL mutation was found in 10% cases while Protein S deficiency was detected in 2.7% cases [56].

IMMUNOLOGIC SCREEN

The association of recurrent losses of natural or artificial pregnancies with immunologic abnormalities has been termed as *immunologic recurrent abortion* (IRA) when other factors such as anatomical abnormalities, endocrine disorders, and abnormal karyotypes have been ruled out. The following immunologic components were studied:

1. *Natural killer (NK) cells*: NK cells are the predominant leukocytes of the endometrium during the implantation phase and early pregnancy. They modulate trophoblastic invasion and angiogenesis. Higher NK cell proportions are prone to implantation defects and pregnancy failures [57,58].
2. *Helper T cells (T_H)*: For maintenance of pregnancy, there should be balance between T_H1/T_H2 cells, with T_H2 lymphocytic predominance, and a stable interplay with interleukins and NK cells. In the absence of such milieu, there is augmented cytotoxic activity of trophoblasts that leads to pregnancy loss in the first trimester [57,58].
3. *Leptin*: Leptin is a cytokine-like hormone with pleiotropic effect in modulating immune responses. It activates and stimulates monocytes, dendritic cells, and macrophages to produce T_H1-type and proinflammatory cytokines like IFN-γ and interleukin (IL)-2 and modulate adaptive immunity. Serum leptin levels are higher in RPL secondary to immunologic or unexplained causes [58].
4. *Increased levels of serum cytokines* measured by Milliplex Luminex with XMAP (Multianalyte profiling) technology in women with RPL compared to normal pregnant women suggests their possible role for miscarriage. Cytokines like tumor necrosis factor (TNF)-α, IFN-γ, and IL-8 are increased and IL-6 decreased significantly ($p < .001$) in the RPL group compared to control. There was no significant correlation between cytokines and FSH and LH, whereas IFN-γ was strongly correlated with LH and prolactin in the miscarriage group [59,60].

However, testing for human leukocyte antigen (HLA), anti-HY antibodies, NK cell, or cytokine levels is not routinely recommended. Immunologic treatments previously practiced like lymphocyte immune therapy or paternal leukocyte immunization, intravenous immunoglobulins, third-party donor cell immunization, or membrane infusions of trophoblasts are not recommended except for research purposes [59,60].

Infections

High-grade fever secondary to any infection in pregnancy usually leads to index pregnancy loss rather than recurrent abortions. However, infections that recur or have a relapsing and remitting course may cause miscarriage in subsequent pregnancy. Unless the patient shows signs or symptoms of a particular disease, routine screening or follow-up for antibody titers for all infections is not recommended. Mycoplasma, ureaplasma, *Toxoplasma gondii*, *Chlamydia trachomatis*, cytomegalovirus, *Listeria monocytogenes*, rubella, herpes simplex virus (HSV), measles, and coxsackie viruses, may cause first-trimester abortions by infecting the endometrium, endocervix, or the fetoplacental unit [2].

In endometritis, a molecular marker for endometrial health called nCyclinE, which is a glandular epithelial nuclear cyclin, is raised. Abnormally high levels of this marker indicate that the pregnancy is likely to fail, while normal levels suggest that it is likely to succeed.

Platelet counts rise with infections or inflammations and act as acute-phase reactants. Mete Ural et al. found that platelet count and platelet distribution width increased in women with RPL. Thus, platelet indices are cost-effective, easy to measure, easily available, and practical markers for the prediction of RPL [61,62].

Psychological factors

RPL will cause psychological trauma to affected couples, and women, especially, are susceptible to psychosomatic disorders including depression, anxiety, and feelings of incompleteness and guilt. A possible psychological association for RPL was suggested in various studies. In a study that compared two groups of RPL couples, the cohort that received tender care apart from the routine obstetric care had significantly higher (more than twice) live birth rates as compared to the cohort receiving only routine obstetric care [63].

Unexplained RPL

Despite extensive workup, the cause for RPL is not found in up to 50% of cases, and these are categorized as unexplained RPL or unexplained recurrent abortion (URA). Plausible immunologic factors like dysregulated NK-cell activity, the presence of cytotoxic antibodies, the lack of maternal blocking antibodies, and an inherent tendency for augmented inflammatory response are attributed as causative hypotheses [13,14]. These factors either alone or as a multitude may be responsible for RPL. No specific investigation is recommended to measure immunologic factors, and only prenatal counseling and continuous monitoring are advised to manage unexplained cases of RPL.

ROLE OF PROGESTERONE IN RPL

Progesterone hormone is essential for implantation and continuation of pregnancy. It has an immunomodulatory action and shifts the balance to the T_H2 cytokine response, which has an anti-inflammatory role and supports pregnancy [64]. It stabilizes the endometrium, is required for embryo implantation, and plays a pivotal role in various immune responses for preparing a milieu so as to sustain the pregnancy. Thus, a deficiency of progesterone probably causes abortions. Various synthetic and natural progesterones are available and can be used by oral, vaginal, and parenteral routes. Efficacy of a specific dose or specific route over the other is not proven; however, higher doses are used in assisted reproduction as compared to spontaneous conceptions, especially in the first trimester [65].

Literature in the recent past suggested positive results with the use of progesterone in RPL. However, after the release of the Progesterone in Women with Unexplained Recurrent Miscarriage (PROMISE) trial, a randomized controlled trial (RCT) involving 1568 patients, the conclusion was that treatment by progesterone in the first trimester has no improved outcomes in women with unexplained RPL. Progesterone therapy if already started can be continued, explaining limited or unproven benefit of such treatment to the couple [66]. From our clinical experience, we prefer supplementing progesterone in high-risk pregnancies,

especially in stimulated cycles provided there are no contraindications for their use.

PRISM trial The Progesterone in Spontaneous Miscarriage (PRISM) trial evaluated if progesterone treatment for women with early pregnancy bleeding results in a higher incidence of live births than placebo treatment. It is a double-blinded, placebo-controlled RCT. Eligible participants were between 16 and 39 years old, had completed 12 weeks or less of pregnancy, presented with vaginal bleeding, and had an intrauterine gestational sac visible on ultrasound. Women treated with progesterone experienced similar rates of live birth as those treated with placebo. Adverse outcomes were similar between both groups [67].

OTHER AVAILABLE TREATMENT OPTIONS OF DOUBTFUL ROLES

1. Anticoagulation therapy does not improve the pregnancy outcome in nonthrombophilic women with unexplained RPL [68].
2. TNF-α inhibitors and granulocyte colony-stimulating factors (G-CSFs) are under trials for treatment of patients with unexplained RPL.
3. Corticosteroids or intravenous immunoglobulin therapy are yet unproven for RPL.

MANAGEMENT

There is no fixed/definitive protocol to treat couples with RPL; as it can be multifactorial, a combination of therapies tailored for the individual patient needs to be applied. Couples should be reassured that even if the cause is not identified after a multitude of investigations, 60%–65% of couples will have a favorable pregnancy outcome. Treatment should be specific if the cause is identified, otherwise general supportive measures are necessary for optimal perinatal outcome (Table 1.4).

CONCLUSION

- The cause for RPL may be multifactorial, and when a definite cause is identified, correcting the underlying cause improves the outcome. Workup for RPL should be initiated after two losses and early in those with fertility issues.
- Even in unexplained RPL, with a higher number of abortions, such as three or four, the probability of carrying the next pregnancy to term is

Table 1.4 General advice to patients with recurrent first-trimester abortions

Participate in preconceptional genetic counseling

Take periconceptional folic acid

Avoid modifiable risk factors: smoking, alcohol, excessive caffeine

Maintain average BMI, avoid vigorous exercise in periconceptional period

Get involved in healthy recreational activities to reduce stress and other anxiety disorders

Note that treatment with antioxidants or multivitamins for men did not show any superior effect

Ensure surveillance and regular follow-up in RPL clinics

Recommend anti-D injections if mother is Rh negative and partner is Rh positive

Women who had first-trimester miscarriage do not need to delay their next conception except if medically indicated. Women who conceived within 6 months of abortion had good pregnancy outcomes as compared to women who took longer periods to conceive

Source: From Nybo Andersen AM et al., *BMJ.* 2000; 320:1708–12.

60%–70%, which is higher than the probability of losing the next pregnancy.

- Though women with RPL are categorized as high-risk pregnancies, a detailed history and clinical examination, evidence-based workup, genetic counseling, psychological support, and reassurance are cornerstones for a favorable outcome in RPL.

POINTS TO PONDER

- Despite extensive studies and research, pregnancy outcomes in women with RPL to date remain unknown to the treating physician and the couples. Positive counseling, tender care, and regular follow-up in RPL clinics provide the best outcomes.
- Further research into the entity being labeled as unexplained RPL is required to reduce the economic burden incurred following investigations and treatment of women with RPL.
- Overtreatment of RPL without justifiable evidence should be avoided.

REFERENCES

1. Stirrat GM. Recurrent miscarriages. *Lancet.* 1990;336:673–5.
2. Rohilla M, Muthyala T. Recurrent Pregnancy Loss (RPL)—Causes and management. *J Gynecol Neonatal Biol.* 2017;3(2):5–8.
3. Rasmark Roepke E, Matthiesen L, Rylance R, Christiansen OB. Is the incidence of recurrent pregnancy loss increasing? A retrospective register-based study in Sweden. *Acta Obstet Gynecol Scand.* 2017;96: 1365–72.
4. Nastaran F, Marcelle I, Cedars , Heather G, Huddleston HG. Cost-effectiveness of cytogenetic evaluation of products of conception in the patient with a second pregnancy loss. *Fertil Steril.* 2012;98(1):151–5.
5. World Health Organization. *International Classification of Disease*; 2000.
6. Kolte AM, Bernardi LA, Christiansen OB et al. ESHRE special interest group, early pregnancy. Terminology for pregnancy loss prior to viability: A consensus statement from the ESHRE early pregnancy special interest group. *Hum Reprod.* 2015;30(3):495–98.
7. Royal College of Obstetricians and Gynaecologists. *The Investigation and Treatment of Couples with Recurrent First-Trimester and Second-Trimester Miscarriage*; 2011. GTG No. 17.
8. Practice Committee of the American Society for Reproductive Medicine. Evaluation and treatment of recurrent pregnancy loss: A committee opinion. *Fertil Steril.* 2012;98(5):1103–11.
9. Silver RM, Branch DW, Goldenberg R, Iams JD, Klebanoff MA. Nomenclature for pregnancy outcomes: Time for a change. *Obstet Gynecol.* 2011;118(6):1402–8.
10. Kutteh WH. Novel strategies for the management of recurrent pregnancy loss. *Semin Reprod Med.* 2015;33(3):161–8.
11. Egerup P, Kolte AM, Larsen EC, Krog M, Nielsen HS, Christiansen OB. Recurrent pregnancy loss: What is the impact of consecutive versus nonconsecutive losses? *Hum Reprod.* 2016;31:2428–34.
12. Nybo Andersen AM, Wohlfahrt J, Christens P, Olsen J, Melbye M. Maternal age and fetal loss: Population based register linkage study. *BMJ* 2000;320:1708–12.

13. Holly B, Danny J. Recurrent pregnancy loss: Etiology, diagnosis, and therapy. *Rev Obstet Gynecol.* 2009;2(2):76–83.

14. Bhattacharya S, Townend J, Shetty A, Campbell D, Bhattacharya S. Does miscarriage in an initial pregnancy lead to adverse obstetric and perinatal outcomes in the next continuing pregnancy? *BJOG* 2008;115:1623–29.

15. Hammoud AO, Merhi ZO, Diamond M, Baumann P. Recurrent pregnancy loss and obstetric outcome. *Int J Gynecol Obstet* 2007;96:28–9.

16. Landres IV, Milki AA, Lathi RB. *Hum Reprod.* 2010;25:1123–6.

17. Fariello RM, Pariz JR, Spaine DM et al. Association between obesity and alteration of sperm DNA integrity and mitochondrial activity. *BJU Int.* 2012;110:863–7.

18. Carrell DT, Liu L, Peterson CM et al. Sperm DNA fragmentation is increased in couples with unexplained recurrent pregnancy loss. *Arch Androl.* 2003;49(1):49–55.

19. De Fleurian G, Perrin J, Ecochard R et al. Occupational exposures obtained by questionnaire in clinical practice and their association with semen quality. *J Androl.* 2009;30(5):566–79.

20. Martenies SE, Perry MJ. Environmental and occupational pesticide exposure and human sperm parameters: A systematic review. *Toxicology.* 2013;307(10):66–73.

21. Rittenberg V, Sobaleva S, Ahmad A et al. Influence of BMI on risk of miscarriage after single blastocyst transfer. *Hum Reprod.* 2011;26:2642–50.

22. Boots C, Stephenson MD. Does obesity increase the risk of miscarriage in spontaneous conception? *Semin Reprod Med.* 2011;29:507–13.

23. Rasch V. Cigarette, alcohol, and caffeine consumption: risk factors for spontaneous abortion. *Acta Obstet Gynecol Scand.* 2003;82:182–8.

24. Cnattingius S, Signorello LB, Anneren G et al. Caffeine intake and the risk of first-trimester spontaneous abortion. *N Engl J Med.* 2000;343:1839–45.

25. Plana-Ripoll O, Parner E, Olsen J, Li J. Severe stress following bereavement during pregnancy and risk of pregnancy loss: Results from a population based cohort study. *J Epidemiol Community Health.* 2016;70:424–9.

26. Hyde KJ, Schust DJ. Genetic considerations in recurrent pregnancy loss. *Cold Spring Harb Perspect Med.* 2015;5:a023119.

27. Benkhalifa M, Kasakyan S, Clement P et al. Array comparative genomic hybridization profiling of first-trimester spontaneous abortions that fail to grow in vitro. *Prenatal Diagn.* 2005;25:894–900.

28. Bernardi LA, Plunkett BA, Stephenson MD. Is chromosome testing of the second miscarriage cost saving? A decision analysis of selective versus universal recurrent pregnancy loss evaluation. *Fertil Steril.* 2012;98:156–61.

29. Carp H, Guetta E, Dorf H, Soriano D, Barkai G, Schiff E. Embryonic karyotype in recurrent miscarriage with parental karyotypic aberrations. *Fertil Steril.* 2006;85:446–50.

30. Gleicher N, Barad DH. A review of and commentary on the ongoing second clinical introduction of preimplantation genetic screening (PGS) to routine IVF practice. *J Assist Reprod Genet.* 2012;12:1159–66.

31. Gleicher N, Kushnir VA, Barad DH. Preimplantation genetic screening (PGS) still in search of a clinical application: A systematic review. *Reprod Biol Endocrinol.* 2014;12:22.

32. Romero ST, Sharshiner R, Stoddard GJ, Ware Branch D, Silver RM. Correlation of serum fructosamine and recurrent pregnancy loss: Case-control study. *J Obstet Gynaecol Res.* 2016;42(7):763–8.

33. American Diabetes Association. Standards of medical care in diabetes. *Diabetes Care.* 2016;391(1):S1–S106.

34. Lois J, Knopp RH, Kim H et al. Elevated pregnancy losses at high and low extremes of maternal glucose in early normal and diabetic pregnancy. *Diabetes Care.* 2005;28:1113–7.

35. Salker MS, Singh Y, Zeng N, Chen H, Zhang S, Umbach AT. Loss of endometrial sodium glucose cotransporter SGLT1 is detrimental to embryo survival and fetal growth in pregnancy. *Sci Rep.* 2017;7(1):12612.

36. Lazarus J, Brown RS, Daumerie C, Hubalewska-Dydejczyk A, Negro R, Vaidya B. European thyroid association guidelines for the management of subclinical hypothyroidism in pregnancy and in children. *Eur Thyroid J.* 2014;3:76–94.

37. Alexander EK, Pearce EN, Brent GA et al. Guidelines of the American Thyroid Association for the diagnosis and management of thyroid disease during pregnancy and the postpartum. *Thyroid*. 2017;27:315–89.

38. Kalra S, Agarwal S, Aggarwal R, Ranabir S. Trimester-specific thyroid-stimulating hormone: An Indian perspective. *Indian J Endocr Metab*. 2018;22:1–4.

39. The TABLET Trial: A Randomised Controlled Trial of the Efficacy and Mechanism of Levothyroxine Treatment on Pregnancy and Neonatal Outcomes in Women with Thyroid Antibodies; 2012.

40. Bliddal S, Nielsen HS, Krogh-Rasmussen A et al. Thyroid peroxidase antibodies do not predict outcome in 900 women with recurrent pregnancy loss. *Endocr Abstr*. 2017;49:OC13.2.

41. Van den Boogaard E, Vissenberg R, Land JA et al. Significance of (sub)clinical thyroid dysfunction and thyroid autoimmunity before conception and in early pregnancy: A systematic review. *Hum Reprod Update*. 2011;17:605–19.

42. Kim NY, Cho HJ, Kim HY et al. Thyroid autoimmunity and its association with cellular and humoral immunity in women with reproductive failures. *Am J Reprod Immunol*. 2011;65:78–87.

43. Alexander EK, Pearce EN, Brent GA et al. Diagnosis and management of thyroid disease during pregnancy and the postpartum. *Thyroid*. 2017;27(3).

44. Lata K, Dutta P, Sridhar S, Rohilla M, Srinivasan A, Prashad G, Shah V, Bhansal A. Thyroid autoimmunity and obstetric outcomes in women with recurrent miscarriage: A case–control study. *Endocr Connect*. 2013;2(2):118–24.

45. Wang Y, Zhao H, Li Y, Zhang J, Tan J, Liu Y. Relationship between recurrent miscarriage and insulin resistance. *Gynecol Obstet Invest*. 2011;72:245–51.

46. Chakraborty P, Goswami SK, Rajani S et al. Recurrent pregnancy loss in polycystic ovary syndrome: Role of hyperhomocysteinemia and insulin resistance. *PLOS ONE*. 2013;8(5):e64446.

47. Celik N, Evsen MS, Sak ME, Soydinc E, Gul T. Evaluation of the relationship between insulin resistance and recurrent pregnancy loss. *Ginekol Pol*. 2011;82:272–5.

48. Jakubowicz DJ, Essah PA, La MS, Jakubowicz S, Baillargeon J-P, Koistinen R. Reduced serum glycodelin and insulin-like growth factor-binding protein-1 in women with polycystic ovary syndrome during first trimester of pregnancy. *J Clin Endocrinol Metab*. 2004;89(2):833–9.

49. Eftekhari N, Mohammadalizadeh S. Pregnancy rate following bromocriptine treatment in infertile women with galactorrhea. *Gynecol Endocrinol*. 2009;25(2):122–4.

50. Ziakas PD, Pavlou M, Voulgarelis M. Heparin treatment in antiphospholipid syndrome with recurrent pregnancy loss: A systematic review and meta-analysis. *Obstet Gynecol*. 2010;115:1256–62.

51. Noura A, Hajera T, Huda A, Amal A, Maha Mohammed A, Mir Naiman A. Identification of serum cytokines as markers in women with recurrent pregnancy loss or miscarriage using MILLIPLEX analysis. *Biomed Res*. 2018;29(18).

52. D'Ippolito S, Marana R, Di Nicuolo F et al. Effect of low molecular weight heparins (LMWHs) on antiphospholipid antibodies (aPL)–mediated inhibition of endometrial angiogenesis. *PLOS ONE*. 2012;7(1):e29660.

53. Ernest JM, Marshburn PB, Kutteh WH. Obstetric antiphospholipid syndrome: An update on pathophysiology and management. *Semin Reprod Med*. 2011;29:522–39.

54. Lockwood C, Wendel G. Committee on Practice Bulletins. Practice bulletin no. 124: Inherited thrombophilias in pregnancy. *Obstet Gynecol*. 2011;118(3):730–40.

55. Viser J, Ulander VM, Helmerhorst FM, Lampinen K, Morin-Papunen L, Bloemenkamp KW. Thromboprophylaxis for recurrent miscarriage in women with or without thrombophilia. HABENOX: A randomised multicenter trial. *J Thromb Haemost*. 2010;105:295–301.

56. Kumar N, Ahluwalia J, Das R, Rohilla M, Bose S, Kishan H, Varma N. Inherited thrombophilia profile in patients with recurrent

miscarriages: Experience from a tertiary care center in north India. *Obstet Gynecol Sci.* 2015;58(6):514–7.

57. Lee SK, Na BJ, Kim JY et al. Determination of clinical cellular immune markers in women with recurrent pregnancy loss. *Am J Reprod Immunol.* 2013;70:398–411.

58. Stricker RB, Winger EE. Update on treatment of immunologic abortion with low-dose intravenous immunoglobulin. *Am J Reprod Immunol.* 2005;54(6):390–6.

59. Saeed Z, Haleh S, Afsaneh M et al. Serum leptin levels in women with immunological recurrent abortion. *J Reprod Infertil.* 2010;11(1):47–52.

60. Nielsen HS, Wu F, Aghai Z et al. H-Y antibody titers are increased in unexplained secondary recurrent miscarriage patients and associated with low male:female ratio in subsequent live births. *Hum Reprod.* 2010;25:2745–52.

61. Oner A, Hatice I, Ahmet S, Mehmet IH, Metin I, Furuzan K. Can Plateletcrit be a marker for recurrent pregnancy loss? *Clin Appl Thromb/Hemost.* 2016;22(5):447–52.

62. Mete Ural U, Bayoğlu Tekin Y, Balik G, Kir Şahin F, Colak S. Could platelet distribution width be a predictive marker for unexplained recurrent miscarriage? *Arch Gynecol Obstet.* 2014;290(2):233–6.

63. Mehta S, Anjum D. *Psychological Factors and Stress in RPL*. Singapore: Springer; 2018.

64. Raghupathy R, Al-Mutawa E, Al-Azemi M, Makhseed M, Azizieh F, Szekeres-Bartho J. Progesterone-induced blocking factor (PIBF) modulates cytokine production by lymphocytes from women with recurrent miscarriage or preterm delivery. *J Reprod Immunol.* 2009;80:91–9.

65. Schindler AE, Carp H, Druckmann R et al. European Progestin Club Guidelines for prevention and treatment of threatened or recurrent (habitual) miscarriage with progestogens. *Gynecol Endocrinol.* 2015;31(6):447–9.

66. Haas DM, Hathaway TJ, Ramsey PS. Progestogen for preventing miscarriage in women with recurrent miscarriage of unclear etiology. *Cochrane Database Syst Rev.* 2018;(10):CD003511.

67. Coomarasamy A, Adam JD, Versha C, Hoda H, Middleton LJ. A randomized trial of progesterone in women with bleeding in early pregnancy. *N Engl J Med* 2019;380:1815–24.

68. Pasquier E, de Saint ML, Bohec C et al. Enoxaparin for prevention of unexplained recurrent miscarriage: A multicenter randomized double-blind placebo-controlled trial. *Blood.* 2015;125(14):2200–5.

2

Management of recurrent second-trimester missed abortion

RICHA ARORA AND POOJA SIKKA

INTRODUCTION

Intrauterine fetal demise before 22 weeks' gestation is sometimes referred to as late miscarriage [1]. Recurrent pregnancy loss, second-trimester missed abortion, and late miscarriage are all emotionally traumatic for the expecting mother and her family. The woman suddenly loses her fetus after 12 weeks or more of pregnancy. The fetus is generally genetically normal or else it would have aborted earlier. The placenta is formed and implanted. What happens to the fetus that it ends in a missed abortion? It is as if a live human being has died after sustaining a cardiac arrest. If, unfortunately, when such an event occurs, the treating obstetrician has several responsibilities that require deliberation: how to break the news, what investigations need to be carried out, how to help the woman expel the fetus, when to discuss postabortal contraception, and how to prevent the event from recurring. How to do complete evaluations of such patients is still not clearly defined. Clinical guidelines by many international bodies have been recommended, but clinicians often do not adhere to them. A lot of variation in the investigation and treatment protocols still exists. Multiple studies in the past stressed the endocrine and immunologic pathology behind recurrent pregnancy loss (RPL). Newer studies are focusing on the embryonic and endometrial etiology of RPL. Out of desperation, doctors tend to overevaluate, overdiagnose, and overtreat. However, the management of every patient needs to be individualized based on the history and presence of risk factors.

DEFINITION OF MISSED ABORTION

A missed abortion is a pregnancy in which there is a fetal demise, but the products of conception are not expelled from the uterine cavity spontaneously.

A missed abortion is confirmed if an ultrasound shows any of the following features:

- Disappearance of previously detected embryonic cardiac activity
- Absence of cardiac activity when the fetal crown-rump length is greater than 7 mm
- Absence of fetal pole when the mean sac diameter is greater than 25 mm [2]

Recurrent miscarriage are defined as follows:

- Loss of three or more consecutive pregnancies (Royal College of Obstetricians and Gynaecologists [RCOG]) [3]
- Two or more pregnancy losses (European Society of Human Reproduction and Embryology [ESHRE]) [4]
- Two or more failed clinical pregnancies (American Society for Reproductive Medicine [ASRM]) [5]

Incidence: Second-trimester miscarriage accounts for 4% of pregnancy losses.

EPIDEMIOLOGICAL FACTORS

Maternal age

It has been proven time and again that as the maternal age advances, the recurrence risk of miscarriage also increases, especially beyond 35 years of age. Various causes include an increased risk of chromosomal aberrations and diminishing uterine and ovarian function. Paternal age beyond 40 years has also been implicated in recurrent miscarriages.

Reproductive history

The risk of subsequent miscarriage increases after each adverse pregnancy event. Additionally, couples with a history of subfertility, delayed conception, and obstetric complications like preterm delivery or previous stillbirth are at higher risk of miscarriage.

ETIOLOGY

Among various causes implicated in recurrent second-trimester missed abortions, thrombophilias are the most important cause, not only because of their associated frequency but also because of their pathogenesis and the impact of treatment on successful pregnancy outcome.

Some other factors that may cause recurrent missed abortion include chromosomal abnormalities, immunologic factors, uncontrolled chronic illness, and drug abuse.

Certain conditions like uterine malformations and cervical incompetence are also associated with recurrent second-trimester abortions but not with recurrent missed abortions.

Chromosomal abnormalities

About 24% of pregnancy losses during the second trimester can be attributed to chromosomal abnormalities. The common numerical chromosomal abnormalities include trisomy 13, 18, 21, and monosomy X.

Maternal chronic illness

Uncontrolled maternal diabetes, hypertension, thyroid disorders, and autoimmune disorders like scleroderma are known to be associated with an increased incidence of miscarriages.

Drug abuse

Maternal drug abuse including chronic smoking, alcohol, caffeine, and recreational drugs like cocaine have a dose-dependent effect on the rate of miscarriage, due to their adverse effect on trophoblastic invasion.

Immunologic factors

Women with a history of recurrent miscarriages have a propensity to produce a predominant helper T-cell-1 (T_H1)-type response, while those with normal pregnancy have a T_H2-type response and produce antibodies. Antibodies produced by T_H2 cells protect fetal trophoblast antigens from cytotoxic immune response mediated by maternal T_H1 cells.

Thrombophilic factors

Pregnancy is a procoagulant condition. There is a relative increase in the levels of all clotting factors except factor XI and XII, accompanied by a decrease in anticoagulant levels and an increase in fibrinolytic activity. It is hypothesized that women with recurrent miscarriages have an exaggerated thrombotic response that leads to thrombosis of the uteroplacental vasculature and adverse pregnancy outcomes.

Antiphospholipid syndrome (APS)

APS has been recognized as one of the most imperative and treatable causes of recurrent second-trimester missed abortion with the prevalence rate of 15%. The pregnancy loss rate can be as high as 90% in untreated cases.

In 1975, Nilsson [6] first reported the association between repeated spontaneous abortions and lupus anticoagulants; while Graham Hughes [7], in 1984, linked the presence of anticardiolipin anticoagulants (ACAs) to miscarriages. It is since then that recurrent pregnancy loss has been considered as hallmark of APS.

Pathophysiology

- Activation of various procoagulants
- Inactivation of natural anticoagulants
- Complement activation
- Inhibition of syncytiotrophoblast differentiation
- Increased trophoblast apoptosis and impaired trophoblast invasion [8]
  Placental changes in APS include placental infarction, impaired spiral artery remodeling, and decidual inflammation. There is rarely any evidence of intravascular or intervillous blood clots.

Clinical features of APS

- *Venous thrombosis*: Thromboembolism, thrombophlebitis, livedo reticularis
- *Arterial thrombosis*: Stroke, transient ischemic attack (TIA), myocardial ischemia, Libman-Sacks cardiac vegetations, distal extremity and visceral thrombosis, and gangrene
- *Hematologic*: Thrombocytopenia, autoimmune hemolytic anemia
- *Other*: Neurological manifestations, migraine, epilepsy, renal artery or venous thrombosis, arthritis, arthralgia
- *Pregnancy*: RPL, preeclampsia, fetal death

Specific antiphospholipid antibodies

Lupus anticoagulant (LAC): LAC is a group of antibodies directed against certain phospholipid binding proteins. LAC causes *in vitro* prolongation of prothrombin time and partial thromboplastin time. Thus, LAC is paradoxically a powerful thrombotic agent. LAC better correlates with thrombosis, pregnancy morbidity, and thrombosis in patients with systemic lupus erythematosus (SLE) than does ACA.

Anticardiolipin anticoagulant (ACA): This is made up of antibodies directed against specific phospholipid cardiolipins found in platelets and mitochondrial membranes.

β2-Glycoprotein: This is a phospholipid binding anticoagulant plasma protein that inhibits adenosine diphosphate–induced platelet aggregation and prothrombinase activity within platelets. Antibodies against β2-glycoprotein inhibit its anticoagulant activity and thus promote thrombosis. β2-Glycoprotein is expressed in high concentrations on the syncytiotrophoblastic surface and maternal decidual endothelial cells and is thought to be involved in implantation.

Testing for antiphospholipid syndrome

LAC is measured based on specific coagulation tests like platelet neutralization and the dilute Russell viper venom test. For a patient already on anticoagulants, measurement of LAC is better postponed.

ACA and β2-glycoprotein (classes IgM and IgG) antibodies are tested by enzyme-linked immunosorbent assay (ELISA).

Diagnosis of APS is based on the clinical and laboratory classification criterion also known as revised Sapporo criterion or Sydney criterion, 2006.

CLINICAL CRITERION [9]

1. Vascular thrombosis
   One or more episodes of thrombosis that may involve artery, vein, or a small vessel. Thrombosis must be confirmed with appropriate radiological study or by histopathology (thrombosis without considerable inflammation).
2. Pregnancy morbidity
   a. Three or more spontaneous, consecutive abortions at less than 10 weeks' gestation, not related to maternal anatomical or hormonal abnormalities.
   b. One or more unexplained fetal deaths after 10 weeks or beyond, of a fetus that is morphologically normal (confirmed with ultrasonography or clinical examination after expulsion).
   c. One or more iatrogenic preterm deliveries at less than 34 weeks' gestation of a morphologically normal fetus due to obstetric indications like placental insufficiency, severe preeclampsia, or eclampsia.

LABORATORY CRITERION

The persistent presence of any one or more of these antibodies in plasma or serum, tested twice or more, at least 12 weeks apart, in medium or high titer is required to confirm diagnosis of APS:

1. Lupus anticoagulant (LAC)
2. Anticardiolipin (aCL) antibody (IgM or IgG)
3. Anti-β2-glycoprotein-1 antibody (IgM or IgG)

The International Society on Thrombosis and Hemostasis has instituted guidelines that should be used for the testing of antiphospholipid antibodies.

Medium or high titer is defined as titers greater than 40 MPL/GPL or greater than the 99th percentile.

The presence of at least one clinical and one laboratory criterion is required to diagnose APS.

Risk stratification based on antiphospholipid titers

Low-risk antiphospholipid (aPL): Isolated or transient positive aCL or β2-glycoprotein I antibodies at low or medium titers.

Medium-high aPL: IgG/IgM ACA or IgG/IgM β2-glycoprotein Ab in titers greater than 40 GPL/MPL or greater than the 99th percentile.

High-risk aPL profile: LAC positive, or the presence of two or three positive aPL antibodies in combination.

APS has recently been separated into two different entities

- Thrombotic antiphospholipid syndrome or TAPS
- Antiphospholipid syndrome associated with obstetric morbidity or OAPS, which includes pregnancy morbidity criterion [1]

Certain studies have shown that women who did not fit in the diagnosis of APS due to low titers (less than 40 MPL/GPL or less than the 99th percentile) had outcomes that were comparable to women

with high titers. Some other studies have conflicting results that demonstrate that women with lower titers had good prognoses.

In the PREGNANTS study [10] of 750 singleton pregnancies with primary APS, Saccone et al. concluded that the most common antibody present in APS is ACA, while the lowest birth rates and highest incidence of adverse pregnancy outcomes are associated with anti-β2-glycoprotein. Also, women with more than one antibody have an increased risk of obstetric complications. The probability of successful pregnancy in women with triple-positive antibodies is nearly 30%.

Other thrombophilias

Inherited thrombophilias include:

- Activated protein C resistance
- Factor V Leiden mutation
- Protein C/S deficiency
- Antithrombin III deficiency
- Hyperhomocysteinemia
- Prothrombin gene mutation

These thrombophilias are well-known causes of systemic thrombosis. They have also been implicated as a possible cause of thrombosis of uteroplacental circulation leading to recurrent miscarriages and late pregnancy complications.

A meta-analysis [11] of 31 studies suggested that the type of fetal loss varied according to the type of thrombophilia. Factor V Leiden was found to be associated with recurrent first-trimester loss and fetal loss after 22 weeks. Also, an association has been suggested between the presence of activated protein C resistance and the prothrombin gene mutation with recurrent first-trimester miscarriages. In an observational study from the northern part of India, Kumar et al. investigated inherited thrombophilia in women with recurrent miscarriages. A total of 12.5% (5/40) patients had an abnormality in inherited thrombophilia profile. Heterozygous FVL mutation was found in 10% cases, while protein S deficiency was detected in 2.7% cases. The frequency of FVL mutation in RM cases in different population and countries varies from 3% to 40%. Among the Indian population, the frequency ranges from 2.3% to 5% [12].

The therapeutic role of anticoagulants in women with a history of recurrent missed abortion with inherited thrombophilia but no past history of thrombosis remains inconclusive. Various studies, like, the LIVE-ENOX study, HepASA Trial, and ALIFE failed to improve pregnancy outcome with antithrombotic prophylaxis. However, a few cohort studies report possible beneficial effects of heparin on live birth rates in these women.

An association between inherited thrombophilias and adverse pregnancy outcome is difficult to establish due to certain facts. First, there is a relatively high prevalence of inherited thrombophilias among asymptomatic patients. Second, various cohort studies have failed to establish any strong association between thrombophilias and adverse pregnancy outcomes; there is also a lack of data suggesting any favorable outcomes despite treatment or intervention.

MANAGEMENT

Even though many studies have reported successful pregnancies in women with APS without treatment, the incidence of complications is quite high. During pregnancy, the concentration of all clotting factors except factor XI and XII increases. In a pregnant woman with APS, this hypercoagulable state due to increased level of coagulation factors, plasminogen activator inhibitors, and activated protein C resistance with decreased protein S activity can cause threatening complications for both the fetus and the mother.

Therefore, management of these women should include:

- Assessment of risk factors
- Preconceptional counseling

History

- Obstetric history: Miscarriages, stillbirth, preterm deliveries, preeclampsia, successful pregnancies
- Medical history: Autoimmune diseases, APS, thrombophilic disorders, toxins, drugs
- Family history: History of thrombosis, transient ischemic attack, cerebrovascular accident, recurrent pregnancy losses

Physical examination

- Signs of endocrine, gynecological disease, or autoimmune disease
- Opportunity to screen: Pap smear for cervical cancer, thallasemia testing, immunization for rubella, varicella, hepatitis B vaccine

Investigations

- Antiphospholipid antibodies
- Thrombophilia screen (only if personal or family history of thrombosis, or in research setting)
- Blood glucose
- Thyroid function test

Counseling: Psychological support, risk of recurrence, available treatment options

Prepregnancy: Optimize medical conditions, start aspirin and folic acid

Subsequent pregnancy: Psychological support, heparin, serial ultrasonography monitoring

Third trimester: Fetal and maternal surveillance: preeclampsia, placental insufficiency, fetal growth restriction

Postpartum: Continue thromboprophylaxis for 6 weeks postpartum

Consider long-term aspirin prophylaxis

Figure 2.1 Approach to the patient with recurrent second-trimester missed abortions.

- Individualization of the treatment plan
- Careful pregnancy surveillance

Women should ideally be referred to a center for specialist maternal care. Testing should be done from reliable laboratory services with quality assurance. Multidisciplinary support by departments like hematology, rheumatology, and radiology should be easily assessable for these women (Figure 2.1).

Assessment of risk factors

Well-established history-based predictive factors include

- Pregnancy morbidity
- Thrombosis
- Presence of SLE and other autoimmune diseases

Laboratory findings linked with adverse pregnancy outcomes include:

- Presence of more than one aPL antibody
- LAC positive
- Hypocomplementemia
- False-positive cytomegalovirus IgM
- Triple positivity (presence of all-LAC, ACA, and β2-glycoprotein antibody in medium to high titers) has been proven to be the most significant risk factor [13]

Preconceptional counseling

- Folic acid supplementation
- Initiation of low-dose aspirin [13]
- Optimization of medical health and drugs before conception

Treatment during pregnancy

Aim: To reduce the risk of thrombosis, miscarriage, placental insufficiency, preeclampsia, iatrogenic preterm delivery, and stillbirth. The likelihood of a successful pregnancy in women with APS exceeds 70% when treated properly.

The current treatment includes low-dose aspirin (75–100 mg/day) and heparin (unfractionated or low molecular weight) [14]. This recommendation is based on the results from two randomized controlled trials that compared the efficacy of aspirin alone and aspirin in combination with heparin. A

Cochrane review published in 2005 also concluded that women with recurrent miscarriages and APS be treated with combined low-dose aspirin and heparin [15].

Ideally, aspirin is started preconceptionally because of its probable favorable effect on implantation. Heparin is started after confirming intrauterine pregnancy. A baseline platelet count should be assessed prior to starting treatment. Low molecular weight heparin may be preferred over unfractionated heparin since it is easier to administer. The dose of heparin depends on the patient's history and aPL profile.

Suggested heparin regimes for APS in pregnancy are as follows [16]:

- APS without prior thrombosis
  - *Recurrent early miscarriage—prophylactic dose*
    - *Unfractionated heparin*: 5000–7500 U subcutaneously (SC), 12 hourly
    - *Low molecular weight heparin (LMWH)*: Enoxaparin 40 mg SC, once a day/30 mg SC, 12 hourly
    - *Dalteparin*: 5000 U, SC, once or twice a day
  - *Fetal death beyond 10 weeks or prior preterm delivery at less than 34 weeks due to uteroplacental insufficiency or preeclampsia)—therapeutic dose*
    - *Unfractionated heparin*: 7500–10,000 U SC, 12 hourly in the first trimester and 10,000 U SC, 12 hourly in second and third trimesters
    - *LMWH*: Enoxaparin 30 mg SC, 12 hourly
    - *Dalteparin*: 5000 U, SC, 12 hourly
- APS with thrombosis—*therapeutic dose*
  - *Unfractionated heparin*: 8–12 hourly, adjusted to maintain activated partial thromboplastin time (aPTT) in therapeutic range
  - *LMWH*: Enoxaparin 1 mg/kg SC, twice daily, or dalteparin, 200 U/kg, SC, twice daily with monitoring of anti-Xa activity

---

Rarely, a woman may present with a positive aPL antibody (laboratory criteria) but does not have any thrombotic or obstetric criteria. Such a woman does not actually fall in the definition of APS and pose a clinical dilemma. A woman in this situation may be considered for low-dose aspirin during pregnancy and the postpartum period.

REFRACTORY OBSTETRIC APS

APS-related pregnancy morbidity includes recurrent first-trimester miscarriages, missed abortion or stillbirth in the second and third trimesters, and early-onset or severe preeclampsia. Other complications that may be seen in women with aPL include recurrent implantation failure, placental abruption and hematomas [13].

Even despite recommended treatment with aspirin and heparin, approximately 20% of women suffering from OAPS fail to achieve a successful live birth. These cases with recurrent adverse obstetric outcomes like fetal death or extreme preterm birth due to uteroplacental insufficiency or severe preeclampsia, despite adequate treatment with low-dose aspirin and heparin, are referred to as refractory OAPS. Little evidence is available to guide treatment in these cases.

Various therapies that have been tried in refractory OAPS include:

- *Corticosteroids*: Prednisolone, 10 mg/day up to 14 weeks
- Intravenous immunoglobulin (IVIG)/plasma exchange
- Hydroxychloroquine
- *Statins*: Pravastatin, 20 mg/day, in cases of severe placental insufficiency with preeclampsia (to be started when placental insufficiency is detected)
- *Tumor necrosis factor inhibitor*: Etanercept

However, data regarding their efficacy and safety in pregnancy are lacking.

CATASTROPHIC ANTIPHOSPHOLIPID SYNDROME

Catastrophic antiphospholipid syndrome (CAPS) is an infrequent but most severe thrombotic presentation of APS. The international consensus statement for classification criteria includes the following:

- Clinically evident thrombosis of three or more organs or systems

- Rapid disease progression of disease pathology, over less than a week
- Histopathological confirmation of thrombosis in at least one organ
- Positive serology for aPL

Precipitating factors include discontinuation of anticoagulation in a known case of APS, surgical intervention, or infection. The incidence of CAPS during pregnancy or puerperium is about 5%–6%. The mortality rate is very high due to the fulminant course of the disease.

Management includes combination therapy with glucocorticoids, heparin, plasma exchange, and IVIG [9].

PREGNANCY COMPLICATIONS AND SURVEILLANCE

Women with APS are at increased risk of developing placental insufficiency and preeclampsia. Serial ultrasounds to assess fetal growth are recommended. Surveillance with nonstress test or biophysical profile should begin at 32 weeks in the absence of any other obstetrical complication. The presence of fetal growth restriction or maternal hypertension may require early and more frequent fetal surveillance.

POSTPARTUM THROMBOPROPHYLAXIS

Postpartum thromboprophylaxis should be strongly considered in all women with APS and is absolutely indicated in women with prior thrombosis. Treatment is usually continued until 6 weeks postpartum. Unfractionated heparin, LMWH, and warfarin are all safe for breastfeeding mothers. Recent data suggest that long-term low-dose aspirin may decrease the lifetime risk of thrombosis in these women [9].

Any kind of pregnancy loss or adverse pregnancy outcome causes significant emotional grief, despair, and apprehension in a couple. This becomes worse as the number of miscarriages increases. Even after detailed evaluation of all causes, more than a third of cases remain unexplained. Such couples not only need comprehensive evaluation but also hope and compassionate care.

REFERENCES

1. Antovic A, Sennström M, Bremme K, Svenungsson E. Obstetric antiphospholipid syndrome. *Lupus Sci Med*. 2018;5(1):e000197.
2. Stamatopoulos N, Condous G. Ultrasound follow-up in the first trimester when pregnancy viability is uncertain. *Australas J Ultrasound Med*. 2017;20(3):95–6.
3. Royal College of Obstetricians and Gynaecologists. *The Investigation and Treatment of Couples with Recurrent First-Trimester and Second-Trimester Miscarriage*. 2011. Greentop Guideline No. 17.
4. European Society of Human Reproduction and Embryology, Early Pregnancy Guideline Development Group. *Recurrent Pregnancy Loss*; November 2017.
5. Evaluation and treatment of recurrent pregnancy loss: A committee opinion. *Fertil Steril*. 2012;98(5):1103–11.
6. Nilsson IM, Astedt B, Hedner U, Berezin D. Intrauterine death and circulating anticoagulant ("antithromboplastin"). *Acta Med Scand*. 1975;197(3):153–9.
7. Hughes GRV. Connective tissue disease and the skin. *Clin Exp Dermatol*. 1984; 9:535–44.
8. Cunningham FG, editor. *Williams Obstetrics*. 25th ed. New York, NY: McGraw-Hill; 2018.
9. Tektonidou M, Andreoli L, Limper M et al. EULAR recommendations for the management of antiphospholipid syndrome in adults. *Ann Rheum Dis*. 2019 Oct;78(10):1296–1304.
10. Liu L, Sun D. Pregnancy outcomes in patients with primary antiphospholipid syndrome: A systematic review and meta-analysis. *Medicine*. 2019;98(20).
11. Rey E, Kahn SR, David M, Shrier I. Thrombophilic disorders and fetal loss: A meta-analysis. *Lancet*. 2003;361(9361):901–8.
12. Kumar N, Ahluwalia J, Das R, Rohilla M, Bose S, Kishan H, Varma N. Inherited thrombophilia profile in patients with recurrent miscarriages: Experience from a tertiary care center in north India. *Obstet Gynecol Sci*. 2015;58(6):514–517.
13. De Carolis S, Tabacco S, Rizzo F et al. Antiphospholipid syndrome: An update on risk factors for pregnancy outcome. *Autoimmun Rev*. 2018;17(10):956–66.
14. Abdel-Qader, A., Hassan, F., Mohammad, M. Low-molecular-weight heparin versus unfractioned heparin in pregnant women with recurrent abortion associated with antiphospholipid syndrome. *Egypt J Hosp Med*. 2018:73(5):6616–20.
15. Empson M, Lassere M, Craig J, Scott J. Prevention of recurrent miscarriage for women with antiphospholipid antibody or lupus anticoagulant. *Cochrane Database Syst Rev*. 2005 Apr 18;(2):CD002859.
16. James D, Steer P, Weiner C, Gonik B. *High Risk Pregnancy: Management Options*. 4th ed. St. Louis, MO: Elsevier Saunders; 2011.

3

Approach to one or more second-trimester painless abortions

KG AMULYA AND MINAKSHI ROHILLA

INTRODUCTION

Recurrent pregnancy loss (RPL) is defined as three or more consecutive pregnancy losses before 24 weeks of gestation [1]. The American Society for Reproductive Medicine (ASRM) [2] and the European Society of Human Reproduction and Embryology (ESHRE) [3] define RPL as two or more clinical and consecutive pregnancy losses, excluding ectopic and molar pregnancies. RPL mainly refers to first-trimester abortions, which are more common. The mid-trimester of pregnancy, rightly perceived as the time of the least pregnancy complications, about 3% need more evaluation [4]. This chapter describes the significance and thorough evaluation of patients with one or more mid-trimester losses, specifically, cervical incompetence classically defined as a "painless" abortion.

Cervical insufficiency is characterized by cervical dilatation and shortening at earlier than 37 weeks of gestation in the absence of contractions. It is the progressive cervical dilatation in the late second or early third trimester without contractions, commonly not associated with pain, which results either in prolapse or premature rupture of membranes leading to pregnancy loss or a preterm delivery. Cervical insufficiency is the inability to support pregnancy to term, due to a defect in either the structure or functioning of the cervix.

RISK FACTORS

The computed incidence of cervical insufficiency in the obstetric population is less than 1%. Risk factors for cervical insufficiency include Müllerian anomalies, cervical trauma, and previous obstetric history with one or more mid-trimester losses, when other causes are ruled out [5].

A detailed obstetric history is key for determining a cervical incompetence–related pregnancy loss. A history of recurrent painless pregnancy losses in the second trimester, preterm rupture of membranes at less than 32 weeks, or a previous pregnancy with a documented cervical length of less than 25 mm before the late second trimester are suggestive of insufficiency.

A history of cervical trauma or interventions like therapeutic abortions, cone biopsy, cervical trauma and lacerations, trachelectomy, or maternal connective tissue diseases like Ehlers-Danlos syndrome, where there is a defect in collagen formation of the cervical stroma, are some of the major risk factors leading to cervical insufficiency (Table 3.1). Patients with a history of polycystic

Table 3.1 Risk factors for cervical insufficiency

- Recurrent painless mid-trimester pregnancy losses
- Previous history suggestive of preterm, prelabor rupture of membranes at less than 32 weeks
- Cervical length documented less than 25 mm at less than 27 weeks in a previous pregnancy
- Cervical trauma and interventions like repeated cervical dilatation for therapeutic abortion, cone biopsy, cervical trauma, and lacerations
- Congenital uterine anomalies
- Any connective tissue disorder (e.g., Ehlers-Danlos syndrome)
- Cervical funneling, short cervix, and cervical dilatation in the present pregnancy
- A cervical length of less than 25 mm before 27 weeks of gestation noted at any time in the present pregnancy, even in the absence of cervical funneling
- Polycystic ovary syndrome with insulin resistance

ovary syndrome (PCOS) who present with cervical incompetence exhibit an earlier onset of symptoms and have a worse prognosis of cervical insufficiency [6].

DIAGNOSIS

Assessment of the cervical canal width using a hysterosalpingogram, the ease of insertion of Hegar number 9 dilator with no resistance, the amount of force needed to pull out an inflated Foley catheter along the cervical os, insertion of intracervical Foley catheter, and measurement of force required to stretch the cervix were used as tests for cervical insufficiency by which inconsistent results were derived.

Transvaginal ultrasonogram is widely used as a valid cervical length measurement method that is reproduced easily with a correct method of measurement during the prenatal period in women with significant risk factors. Cervical shortening with cervical length less than 25 mm predicts preterm delivery or mid-trimester loss. Cervical dilatation in the absence of uterine contractions, with

or without rupture of membranes, is diagnostic of cervical insufficiency.

Cervical length measurement

Transvaginal ultrasonogram is performed with the patient in the dorsal lithotomy position. The following factors need to be considered before measuring cervical length [7] (Figure 3.1):

1. Maternal urinary bladder should be empty.
2. Longitudinal aspect of the cervix should be viewed.
3. Cervical canal should be identified.
4. Cervix should be magnified so that it occupies 50%–75% of the screen image.
5. Probe pressure on cervix should be kept to a minimum.
6. Examination should be conducted for a minimum of 3–5 minutes.
7. Measurement is procured by placing calipers at the external and the internal os.

MANAGEMENT

Management of cervical insufficiency [1] depends on various maternal and obstetric factors. It can be either one of the following:

1. Surgical intervention by a cervical cerclage
2. Conservative management

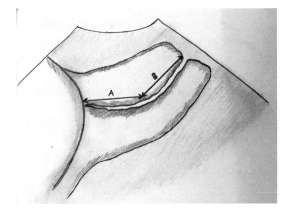

Figure 3.1 Cervical length measurement by transvaginal ultrasonography. Calipers placed at external and internal os. (Cervical length = A + B.)

Indications for a cervical cerclage include clinical history of documented short cervix and/or dilated cervix in index pregnancy and can be allocated to a prophylactic cerclage group (history-indicated or ultrasound-indicated cerclage) and a therapeutic cerclage group (rescue cerclage). A cervical pessary is an alternative to a cerclage procedure; however, the data on pessary are limited with unproven results.

History indicated

This should be provided to women with three or more previous preterm deliveries or in whom the obstetric history is very suggestive of cervical insufficiency. Cerclage is prophylactically performed at around 12–14 weeks of gestation as an elective procedure.

Ultrasound indicated

In a woman with significant risk factors, serial ultrasound monitoring is done. Cerclage is done as a therapeutic procedure in women who screen positive for cervical insufficiency. Ultrasound-indicated cerclage is performed when the cervical length during serial monitoring is less than 25 mm, in less than 24 weeks of gestation, and if there is no herniation of fetal membranes. Sonographic assessment for the cervical length is usually started at 14 weeks of gestation after aneuploidy screening, until 24 weeks of gestation.

With a history of spontaneous preterm delivery or a second-trimester loss, either short cervical length or funneling of the cervix in the absence of a short cervix would prompt an ultrasound-indicated cervical encerclage.

Rescue cerclage

Rescue cerclage is done as a salvage measure when there is cervical dilatation with prolapsing fetal membranes, identified either on clinical examination or by ultrasound in a symptomatic patient. Symptoms such as vaginal discharge, bleeding, or a "pressure" sensation may be present.

The placement of a rescue cerclage should be individualized. The period of gestation at the time of cerclage is the foremost important determinant

to do or undo the procedure. The average gestational age prolonged may be by 5 weeks. A cervix dilated greater than 4 cm or prolapse of fetal membranes beyond the external os predict a high failure rate of cerclage insertion.

Prerequisites for prophylactic cerclage placement

Confirming fetal viability before the procedure is necessary [5] (Table 3.2).

Congenital fetal malformations are excluded. In cases with any increased risk for aneuploidy, the procedure may be delayed until karyotyping is done or an anomaly scan is performed to rule out malformations and aneuploidies.

Screening for any focus of infection, which can predispose the patient for a preterm delivery, should be made.

A urine analysis for any urinary infection and, accordingly, culture and sensitivity of the sample are mandatory. Vaginal swabs to rule out bacterial vaginosis, or swabs for cultures of any infections, should be obtained and treated before a patient is admitted for cerclage. During this screening, cervical length has to be assessed by examination to plan the approach for cerclage, vaginal versus abdominal, especially in women with previous failed cerclage.

In about 50% of women, bacterial invasion of the amniotic membranes is a contributing factor for cervical insufficiency. Amniocentesis for evaluation and treatment of chorioamnionitis before performing a cerclage was not shown to be beneficial and hence is not recommended.

Cervical cerclage is always performed under regional anesthesia and is always preferred over general anesthesia due to lesser-associated risks, unless contraindicated.

Table 3.2 Contraindications to cerclage insertion

- Established preterm labor
- Continuous vaginal bleeding
- Clinical evidence of chorioamnionitis
- Preterm premature rupture of membranes
- Any evidence of compromised fetal status
- Congenital malformation that could be lethal
- Fetal demise

CERCLAGE TECHNIQUES

1. Transvaginal
2. Transabdominal
3. Laparoscopic [5]

Case selection: Transvaginal versus transabdominal cerclage

During screening for infections, an additional assessment of the vaginal portion of cervical length is considered so as to plan the route of encerclage (Figure 3.2). If there is a good portion of cervical length available, then a McDonald encerclage may be planned. If there is a feasible length of vaginal cervix, an option of Shirodkar suture with bladder reflection can be given. The most important indications for transabdominal cerclage are absent vaginal cervix, grossly disrupted cervix, and previous failed vaginal cerclage.

TRANSVAGINAL TECHNIQUES

The two most important techniques of transvaginal cerclage, which are very well known, are the McDonald approach (Figures 3.3 and 3.4) and the Shirodkar approach.

McDonald technique

In the McDonald technique of encerclage, a purse-string suture is inserted as close to the cervicovaginal junction as possible. There is no need to dissect tissue planes. Cervical length remains a good prognostic indicator in this procedure.

Shirodkar procedure

In the Shirodkar approach, anteriorly the bladder and the rectum posteriorly are dissected and separated from the vagina through their respective planes to facilitate the high approach for the placement of the suture. A subepithelial suture is inserted above the cervicovaginal junction close to the internal cervical os.

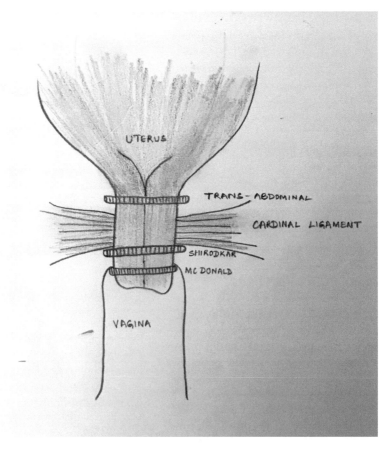

Figure 3.2 The placement of cerclage in different approaches—transabdominal and transvaginal.

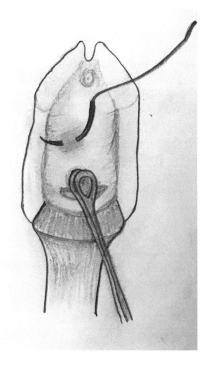

Figure 3.3 The procedure in transvaginal cerclage technique.

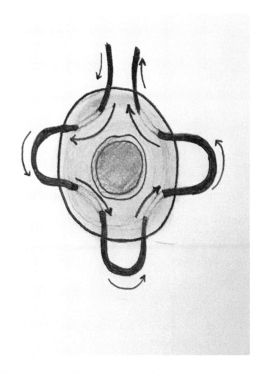

Figure 3.4 McDonald procedure.

Suture materials

Advantages and disadvantages of a particular suture material over another are not reported. The most commonly used sutures are braided Mersilene (Ethicon) tape and Prolene (Ethicon). Mesh can also be used, but there are no data comparing that with the traditional methods. Delayed absorbable sutures are better according to some surgeons, but this requires greater validation.

PROPHYLACTIC TRANSABDOMINAL CERCLAGE

The transabdominal approach is preferred in a woman with a history of cervical incompetence in whom there was a failure of prior vaginal cerclage by an experienced surgeon. It should also be considered in women who have had trachelectomy for gynecological reasons. The abdominal suture may be placed either laparoscopically or by a laparotomy. The laparoscopic techniques are generally preferred in current practice; however, transabdominal methods have higher maternal morbidity than the transvaginal techniques [5].

A Pfannenstiel incision is given and abdominal layers opened. A transverse incision of the vesicouterine peritoneum is performed for bladder retraction. A Mersilene suture through the broad ligament close to the cervical stroma is taken all around, similar to the McDonald stitch, and tied securely.

In the laparoscopic technique, after induction with general anesthesia, a 10 mm primary trocar is inserted supraumbilically. Accessory ports of 5 mm are inserted at a safer site according to the height of the gravid uterus. Laparoscopic cerclage is the replicate of the surgical technique of open surgery, except that routine bladder reflection is not performed, unless it is a case of previous cesarean section. A Mersilene suture is laid down at the isthmic level around the cervix, and the surgical knot is secured.

Women who undergo transabdominal cerclages will undergo regular prenatal follow-up after the procedure. If any need for premature delivery in the case of loss of fetal viability or any maternal complication, cerclage can be removed by either laparotomy or laparoscopically and allowed vaginal delivery or hysterotomy can be performed. Usually, term delivery in women with transabdominal cerclage is performed by a cesarean section.

Transabdominal cerclage can be left *in situ* after delivery by cesarean section for the next pregnancy [8].

Tocolysis, progesterones, and corticosteroids

There are no large randomized trials suggesting routine use of tocolytics [9,10], corticosteroids, or antibiotics [11–13] during a prophylactic cerclage (Figure 3.5). For cerclages placed close to the period of viability of the fetus, corticosteroids may be administered. Similarly, data on progesterone usage in women who have a cerclage *in situ* are limited.

Routine supplementation of progesterone for women with cervical cerclage *in situ* is common in practice, but data do not presently support this approach. Previous studies show a significant hospital admission rate reduction but not in the rate of pregnancy loss [13,14]. Two studies [15,16] indicated that there are no additional benefits with 17-α-hydroxyprogesterone caproate injections for the prevention of preterm delivery in women who had an ultrasound-indicated cerclage.

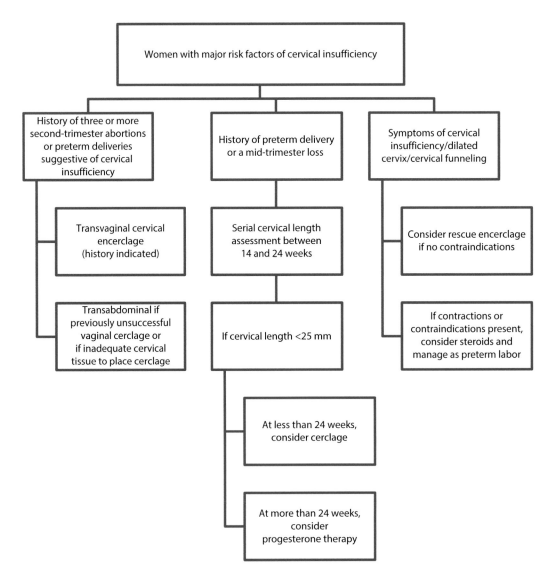

Figure 3.5 Approach to a woman with recurrent mid-trimester abortion or a previous preterm delivery.

There are limited data comparing the systemic and vaginal progesterones used in women with a cervical encerclage *in situ*.

Follow-up

There can be an increase in the cervical length following cerclage, and the immediate cervical assessment following placement of an encerclage may correlate with gestational age at delivery [17–19]. Follow-up by ultrasound after cervical encerclage is not recommended as routine. Regular prenatal follow-up is recommended up to 36 weeks of gestation. Removal of cervical cerclage is done at around 36–38 weeks of gestation. Timing and mode of delivery are decided as per obstetric indication.

Removal of cerclage

If the woman does not go into preterm labor, cervical encerclage is electively removed between 36 and 38 weeks of gestation. It generally requires no anesthesia; if necessary, only short-acting narcotics can be administered intravenously. If any suspicion of chorioamnionitis or established preterm labor arises, emergency removal of the cerclage can be performed. Clear documentation of placement of the knot at the time of cervical cerclage will help in the removal of the cerclage.

SPECIFIC CONDITIONS

Preterm premature rupture of membranes in woman with cerclage *in situ*

A randomized multicenter trial [20] was performed to decide whether to remove or retain cerclage in women who subsequently develop preterm premature rupture of membranes (PPROM). It concluded that there were no statistically significant differences in prolongation of pregnancy by retaining the cerclage after a PPROM. There was a slightly less infectious morbidity with immediate removal of cerclage.

Multiple pregnancy

There are no well-defined guidelines for the treatment of a multiple pregnancy with a short cervical length. Use of progesterones and cervical pessaries as prophylaxis are a few interventions to prevent preterm delivery in a twin pregnancy. Although there are no identifiable benefits of using pessaries, they are beneficial only in selected populations [21].

A multicenter study [22] to test the efficacy of the cervical pessary to reduce the preterm delivery rate in twin gestation and short cervical length was performed. The insertion of a cervical pessary in a twin pregnancy with a short cervical length was associated with a significant reduction in preterm birth.

In a retrospective cohort study [23], a significantly shortened cervical length of less than 15 mm has shown proven benefits from cerclage.

Use of cervical encerclage is not beneficial in all cases but is limited to cases where cervical dilatation is more than 1 cm, where preterm birth of less than 32 weeks was significantly reduced compared to expectant management [24].

REFERENCES

1. Royal College of Obstetricians and Gynaecologists. *The Investigation and Treatment of Couples with Recurrent First-Trimester and Second-Trimester Miscarriage*; 2011. GTG No. 17.
2. American Society for Reproductive Medicine. Evaluation and treatment of recurrent pregnancy loss: A committee opinion. *Fertil Steril.* 2012;98(5):1103–11.
3. Clinical review articles: Recurrent first trimester pregnancy loss. *Obstet Gynaecol Clin North Am.* 2014;41:1–8.
4. Simpson J. Causes of fetal wastage. *Clin Obstet Gynecol.* 2007;50:10–30.
5. Society of Obstetricians and Gynaecologists of Canada. *Cervical Insufficiency and Cervical Cerclage*; February 2019. SOGC clinical practice guideline, No. 373.
6. Wang Y, Gu X, Tao L, Zhao Y. Co-morbidity of cervical incompetence with polycystic ovarian syndrome (PCOS) negatively impacts prognosis: A retrospective analysis of 178 patients. *BMC Pregnancy Childbirth.* 2016; 16(1):308.
7. Kogan KO, Sonek J. How to measure cervical length. *Ultrasound Obstet Gynecol.* 2015;45:358–62.
8. Carter JF, Soper DE. Laparoscopic removal of abdominal cerclage. *JSLS.* 2007;11(3):375–7.

9. Locci M, Nazzaro G, Merenda A et al. Atosiban vs ritodrine used prophylactically with cerclage in ICSI pregnancies to prevent pre-term birth in women identified as being at high risk on the basis of transvaginal ultrasound scan. *J Obstet Gynaecol*. 2006;26:396–401.

10. Visintine J, Airoldi J, Berghella V. Indomethacin administration at the time of ultrasound-indicated cerclage: Is there an association with a reduction in spontaneous preterm birth? *Am J Obstet Gynecol*. 2008;198:643.e1–3.

11. Charles D, Edwards WR. Infectious complications of cervical cerclage. *Am J Obstet Gynecol*. 1981;141:1065–71.

12. Kessler I, Shoham Z, Lancet M et al. Complications associated with genital colonization in pregnancies with and without cerclage. *Int J Gynaecol Obstet*. 1988;27:359–63.

13. Shiffman RL. Continuous low-dose antibiotics and cerclage for recurrent second-trimester pregnancy loss. *J Reprod Med*. 2000;45:323–6.

14. Ayers JW, Peterson EP, Ansbacher R. Early therapy for the incompetent cervix in patients with habitual abortion. *Fertil Steril*. 1982;38:177–81.

15. Berghella V, Figueroa D, Szychowski JM et al. 17α-hydroxyprogesterone caproate for the prevention of preterm birth in women with prior preterm birth and a short cervical length. *Am J Obstet Gynecol*. 2010;202:351.e1–6.

16. Rafael TJ, Mackeen AD, Berghella V. The effect of 17α-hydroxyprogesterone caproate on preterm birth in women with an ultrasound-indicated cerclage. *Am J Perinatol*. 2011;28:389–94.

17. Funai EF, Paidas MJ, Rebarber A et al. Change in cervical length after prophylactic cerclage. *Obstet Gynecol* 1999;94:117–9.

18. Guzman ER, Houlihan C, Vintzileos A et al. The significance of transvaginal ultrasonographic evaluation of the cervix in women treated with emergency cerclage. *Am J Obstet Gynecol*. 1996;175:471–6.

19. Althuisius SM, Dekker GA, van Geijn HP et al. The effect of therapeutic McDonald cerclage on cervical length as assessed by transvaginal ultrasonography. *Am J Obstet Gynecol*. 1999;180:366–9.

20. Galyean A, Garite TJ, Maurel K et al. Removal versus retention of cerclage in preterm premature rupture of membranes: A randomized controlled trial. *Am J Obstet Gynecol*. 2014;211(4):399.e1–7.

21. Huras H, Kalinka J, Dębski R. Short cervix in twin pregnancies: Current state of knowledge and the proposed scheme of treatment. *Ginekol Pol*. 2017;88(11):626–32.

22. Goya M, de la Calle M, Pratcorona L. Cervical pessary to prevent preterm birth in women with twin gestation and sonographic short cervix: A multicenter randomized controlled trial (PECEP-Twins). *Am J Obstet Gynecol*. 2016;214(2):145–52.

23. Roman A, Rochelson B, Fox NS et al. Efficacy of ultrasound-indicated cerclage in twin pregnancies. *Am J Obstet Gynecol*. 2015;212:788.e1–6.

24. Han MN, O'Donnell BE, Maykin MM. The impact of cerclage in twin pregnancies on preterm birth rate before 32 weeks. *J Matern Fetal Neonatal Med*. 2019;32(13):2143–51.

4

Management of pregnancy with recurrent preterm deliveries

SHIVANI SHARMA

INTRODUCTION

Preterm delivery is defined as delivery before 37 completed weeks of pregnancy. It has a long-term effect on a child's well-being, and it is a major determinant of neonatal morbidity and mortality. The incidence of preterm deliveries is 5%–7% in developed countries [1] and is predicted to be much higher in developing nations. The global incidence of preterm birth is around 9.5%, and 85% of them occur in Africa and Asia [2].

The term *recurrent preterm delivery* applies to more than one delivery before 37 completed weeks of gestation. The calculation of accurate gestational age is very important to determine exact gestational age at delivery and to avoid iatrogenic preterm deliveries due to various maternal or fetal indications. The most commonly used tool is calculating gestation from the first day of the last menstrual period (LMP). There are various factors that hinder this calculation, such as menstrual irregularity, some illnesses, amenorrhea due to breastfeeding, and women's recall of her LMP. Similarly, the measurement of fundal height to calculate gestation is also not an accurate method. The best method for calculating gestational age is early ultrasound with fetal anthropometric measurements specific to gestational age. These include measurement of crown rump length before 12 weeks and biparietal diameter and femur length after that, best done before 20 weeks of gestation.

MORBIDITY DUE TO PREMATURITY

With advances in neonatal care, the survival of babies born before term has definitely improved. Morbidity is dependent on birth weight as well as gestational age at the time of delivery, and it has been observed that babies weighing more than 1000 g or born after 28 weeks of pregnancy have better chances of survival. Viability criteria are different in various countries because of the differences in resources and neonatal advanced care facilities. The American College of Obstetricians and Gynecologists (ACOG) [3] recommends that neonatal resuscitation should be done if gestational age is more than 24 weeks but not if it is less than 22 weeks. The Indian Academy of Pediatrics [4] fixed the gestational age at more than 28 weeks to define viability. In a study conducted in England [5], the survival of babies born at 22, 26, and 28 weeks of gestation was 25.4%, 88.2%, and 94.5%, respectively.

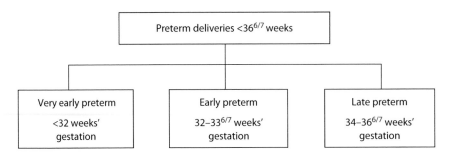

Figure 4.1 Classification of preterm deliveries.

Short-term and long-term complications associated with prematurity

There have been immense improvements in neonatal resuscitation and care, and because of this the overall mortality has declined, but various organ-related dysfunctions persist due to the effects of prematurity. These effects are more severe in infants who are extremely premature according to period of gestation (Figure 4.1). Some of these conditions are short-lived and are manageable with good neonatal intensive care, but some are long-lasting, and studies are still going on to evaluate these effects in later life (Table 4.1).

CAUSE OF RECURRENT PRETERM DELIVERY

There is an interplay of various factors when there is premature cervical dilatation and effacement, which ultimately leads to a baby born before term. It has been seen that there is excessive expression of contraction-associated proteins (CAPs) [7] in conditions causing uterine overdistension. Early activation of placental fetal-uterine cascade and release of maternal corticotrophin-releasing hormones accentuate uterine expression of CAPs and ultimately lead to cervical ripening. In conditions causing maternal stress, premature activation of the fetal placental endocrine axis plays a role in preterm labor.

Table 4.1 Short- and long-term effects of prematurity

System or organ	Short-term complications	Long-term complications
Respiratory system	Respiratory distress syndrome, apnea of prematurity, bronchopulmonary dysplasia	Bronchopulmonary dysplasia, asthma
Cardiovascular	Patent ductus arteriosus, hypotension	Pulmonary hypertension, hypertension in adulthood
Gastrointestinal system	Necrotizing enterocolitis	
Eyes	Retinopathy of prematurity	Retinal detachment, myopia, strabismus
Central nervous system	Short-term neurological injury, intraventricular hemorrhage, periventricular leukomalacia	Cerebral palsy, motor impairment, neurodevelopmental delay, hearing loss
Immunologic	Perinatal sepsis, immune deficiency, hospital-acquired infections	
Hematologic	Anemia, need for transfusions	
Endocrinologic	Hypoglycemia, cortisol deficiency	Insulin resistance, impaired regulation of blood glucose

Source: Patel R. Am J Perinatol. 2016;33(3):318–28.

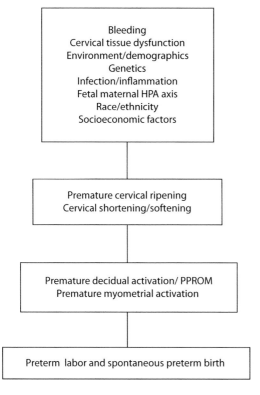

Figure 4.2 Cervical remodeling leading to preterm delivery.

Table 4.2 Risk of recurrent spontaneous preterm birth with outcome of previous pregnancy

First birth outcome	Risk of second delivery less than 35 weeks (%)
Delivery less than 36 weeks	14–15
Term delivery	3

Source: Mazaki-Tovi S et al. Semin Perinatol. 2007;31(3): 142–58.

role in preterm labor. They release membrane metalloproteinases (MMPs), interleukins (IL-6, IL-8), and tumor necrosis factor. All of these lead to activation of labor [7] (Figure 4.2).

Prior preterm birth is an important and independent risk factor for preterm birth. It has been observed that the risk of recurrent preterm birth with a history of one preterm birth is threefold higher. It is further related to the gestation at which previous preterm birth has occurred (Tables 4.2 and 4.3).

The vaginal tract has a specific microbial environment with a predominance of *Lactobacillus* species. It has been observed that in cases of preterm labor, certain microorganisms are found more frequently, such as *Gardnerella vaginalis*, *Fusobacterium* species, *Mycoplasma hominis*, and *Ureaplasma urealyticum* [9]. It is postulated that the invasion of the cervical epithelial barrier by group B streptococcal infection leads to its disruption and ascent of infection by secreting enzyme hyaluronidase [10].

Transplacental, ascending, or retrograde spread of infection into the uterus can lead to inflammation and premature uterine contractions or rupture of membranes. Inflammatory mediators like lipopolysaccharides and cytokines play a pivotal

Table 4.3 Risk factors for preterm delivery

Modifiable	Nonmodifiable
Cocaine or heroin abuse	Previous preterm delivery
Bacterial vaginosis	Black race
Urinary tract infection	History of cervical conization, loop electrosurgical excision procedure
Intrauterine infection	Multifetal pregnancy
Low prepregnancy body mass index ($<18 \text{ kg/m}^2$)	Certain fetal anomalies
Medical disorders like diabetes, hypertension, and thyroid abnormality	Polyhydramnios
Excessive physical work	Short cervix (<25 mm before 28 weeks of pregnancy)
Periodontal diseases	Uterine anomalies
Sexually transmitted infections (chlamydia, gonorrhea, and trichomonas)	Vaginal bleeding
Short pregnancy interval (<18 months)	Iatrogenic

Twin pregnancy and recurrent preterm birth

Women with preterm twin delivery in a prior pregnancy and a single fetus in the next pregnancy are at high risk of preterm delivery. However, risk is not increased if delivery has occurred between 34 and 37 weeks of gestation. Similarly, preterm singleton delivery also increases the risk of preterm delivery in a twin or higher-order pregnancy.

Cervical insufficiency as a cause of recurrent preterm delivery

Cervical insufficiency due to mechanical factors is also an important cause of preterm births. The history of cervical conization, loop electrosurgical excision procedure (LEEP), obstetric injury to the cervix, or intrinsic causes like congenital uterine anomalies and collagen vascular disorder, are important causes of cervical insufficiency.

Previously, digital examination of the cervix was used to determine its length, consistency, effacement, and dilatation to diagnose cervical insufficiency. Transvaginal ultrasonography has now become the gold standard to diagnose incompetent cervix because it is unaffected by maternal obesity, fetal shadowing, or cervical position.

INDICATIONS TO SCREEN FOR TRANSVAGINAL CERVICAL LENGTH

Transvaginal ultrasound for screening of cervical length is indicated in patients with a history of previous spontaneous preterm delivery and singleton pregnancy [11]. Routine screening is not required in women with cervical cerclage, multiple gestation, preterm premature rupture of membranes (PPROM), or placenta previa.

WHEN IT SHOULD BE MONITORED

Cervical length should be assessed between 16 and 24 weeks' gestation; prior to 16 weeks, the lower uterine segment is not developed, so it is difficult to distinguish it from the endocervical canal. Serial ultrasounds should be done every 1–2 weeks until 24 weeks of gestation.

METHOD (CERVICAL LENGTH EDUCATION AND REVIEW PROGRAM: CLEAR)

After the patient has emptied her bladder and is in dorsal recumbent position, gently insert the ultrasound probe into the vagina and guide the probe into the anterior fornix. A sagittal image is obtained occupying two-thirds of the screen such that both internal and external os are seen clearly. Cervical length is measured along the endocervical canal between the internal and external os. Three sets of measurements are taken, and the shortest best means cervical length measurements made keeping laid criterion in consideration and then documenting that length which is the shortest of all and not the mean of 3 measured values. Cervical length less than 25 mm requires intervention.

Recurrent indicated preterm births

These are the births that result due to some complication in the mother or the fetus requiring early termination of pregnancy. The incidence of indicated preterm deliveries is highly variable (1%–5%) and accounts for about one-third of total preterm deliveries. Even a previously indicated preterm delivery is a risk factor for spontaneous recurrent preterm birth (Table 4.4).

Table 4.4 Recurring obstetric conditions requiring early termination of pregnancy

Maternal conditions	Fetal conditions

Hypertensive disorders
    Uncontrolled maternal blood pressure
    Severe preeclampsia, eclampsia
	Severe intrauterine growth retardation

Obstetric hemorrhage
    Placenta previa
    Unexplained vaginal bleeding
    Abruption
	Fetal distress

Prior classical cesarean section	Fetal malformation Previous monochorionic monoamniotic twin pregnancy

Preterm premature rupture of membranes

Symptoms: Patient complains of vaginal passage of colorless, odorless fluid.

Diagnosis: PPROM complicates about 3% of pregnancies and around 30%–40% of preterm deliveries [12].

History: Clear, colorless drainage of fluid vaginally.

Per speculum examination: Pooling of amniotic fluid is seen in vagina or drainage of same is seen through cervical os while coughing.

Ultrasound examination: Document apparent decrease in amniotic fluid volume in a woman with previously documented normal liquor volume.

Vaginal fluid tests:
1. Insulin-like growth factor binding protein
2. Placental α-microglobulin-1
3. Positive fetal fibronectin test (>50 ng/mL)

Amniotic fluid aspiration for culture and sensitivity or Nitrazine tests are not recommended.

Management: Monitor the mother for symptoms of chorioamnionitis by examining her pulse, temperature, presence of lower abdominal pain, vaginal discharge, and reduced fetal movements. For diagnosis of chorioamnionitis, clinical assessment, maternal blood tests (C-reactive protein and white cell count), and fetal heart rate all should be taken into account. These parameters should not be used in isolation.

Offer antibiotics—oral erythromycin 250 mg four times a day for a maximum of 10 days or until labor is established (NICE) (or oral penicillin should be given in patients allergic to erythromycin).

Diagnosis of spontaneous preterm labor with intact membranes

Clinical examination: A woman presents with regular, rhythmic, progressive, and painful contractions leading to dilatation and effacement of cervix. These may be associated with pelvic pressure, menstrual-like cramps, watery vaginal discharge, and low back pain.

Fetal fibronectin test: Fibronectin is a glycoprotein present in maternal blood as well as amniotic fluid. Although the ACOG (2012) does not recommend routine use of the fetal fibronectin test, fibronectin can be detected in cervicovaginal secretions normally before 20 weeks, and if present thereafter, it acts as a marker of possible preterm labor. Women with positive fibronectin test have more risk of spontaneous preterm delivery (28%) compared with those with negative test results (7%). Short cervical length (less than 25 mm) poses a threat of spontaneous delivery before term and when combined with a positive fetal fibronectin test, the risk increases to 64% [11].

PREVENTION OF RECURRENT PRETERM DELIVERY

Progesterone therapy

Progesterone has the most important role in continuation of pregnancy by maintaining myometrial quiescence. It interferes with oxytocin binding, downregulates gap-junction formation, and thus inhibits cervical ripening. It also inhibits apoptosis in fetal membranes and blocks production of cytokines, preventing premature labor. In women with a history of spontaneous preterm delivery, the addition of progesterone therapy prenatally has been found to be beneficial in preventing recurrent preterm delivery. It should be started at 16–20 weeks' gestation and continued until 36 weeks' gestation (Figure 4.3).

Injection hydroxyprogesterone caproate 250 mg intramuscularly given weekly is the treatment of choice [13]. In the case of cervical shortening, micronized progesterone 200–400 mg daily vaginally has been found to be efficacious. Treatment should be started between 16 and 24 weeks of pregnancy and continued at least until 34 weeks' gestation.

Progesterone supplementation has no effect on preterm birth rates in case of multiple pregnancy,

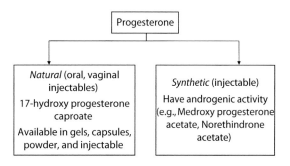

Figure 4.3 Types of progesterone used in prevention of recurrent preterm birth.

PPROM, positive fetal fibronectin test, cervical cerclage stitch in place, or if given after an episode of preterm labor. Progesterone supplementation has been found effective in only one-third of cases of recurrent preterm deliveries.

Tocolytics

Tocolytics usually do not prolong pregnancy duration but are effective in delaying delivery for up to 48 hours. This is useful as it allows transport to facilities where good neonatal care is available. It also provides time for corticosteroids to act.

Nifedipine is the drug of choice in women with preterm labor pains with intact membranes. In conditions where nifedipine is contraindicated, oxytocin receptor antagonists should be used [21]. Betamimetic drugs are best avoided (Table 4.5).

Cervical cerclage and pessary

Cervical cerclage is the placement of suture around the cervix (Figure 4.4).

INDICATIONS AS PER NATIONAL INSTITUTE FOR HEALTH AND CARE EXCELLENCE 2015 GUIDELINES

1. Women found to have a dilated or shortened cervix less than 25 mm during pregnancy on ultrasound done between 16 and 24 weeks of pregnancy (NICE) who have either:
   - Previous preterm prelabor rupture of membranes
   - History of cervical trauma
2. Women with three or more spontaneous second-trimester losses

TIMING

According to the National Institute for Health and Care Excellence (2019), elective cerclage should be performed at 13 to 16 weeks' gestation, after first-trimester screening, nuchal translucency measurement, and fetal evaluation for major congenital malformations. Urgent cervical cerclage should be done in a patient with a history of second-trimester losses attributed to cervical insufficiency after an evaluation of cervical length. Rescue cerclage can be considered in pregnant women between 16 and 27 weeks in case the cervix is dilated and exposed.

CONTRAINDICATIONS

Absolute contraindications include the following:

- Active labor/uterine contractions
- Active vaginal bleeding
- Placental abruption
- Premature rupture of membranes
- Chorioamnionitis/signs of infection

In a high-risk woman with a short cervix, placing a suture around the cervix before or after pregnancy corrects the structural defect in the cervix. In women with a history of one or more preterm deliveries and ultrasound suggestive of cervical length of 25 mm or less, cerclage decreases the chances of preterm delivery to 6.1% from 14% in women on expectant management [15].

The use of preprocedure antibiotics or tocolytics is controversial; they are not recommended and should be used with caution. The cervical stitch should be removed around 36–37 weeks of gestation or earlier if the patient goes into labor or delivery is planned earlier [16].

Cervical pessary

Silicone pessaries in women with cervical length of less than 25 mm at 20–24 weeks of pregnancy have been found to be effective in the prevention of preterm delivery. These pessaries were even used in the case of twin pregnancies, and the average gestation of delivery was found to be higher in women with cervical pessary *in situ* [20].

Role of maternal corticosteroids

Maternal corticosteroids should be considered if gestation is more than 23 weeks, and they must be given after 24 weeks' gestation (American College of Obstetricians and Gynecologists) [17]. A single course of corticosteroids is to be given if delivery is expected within 7 days, including in cases of PPROM or multiple gestation. The recommended use of betamethasone is two doses of 12 mg each, 24 hours apart, and that of dexamethasone is four doses of 6 mg each, every 12 hours. Both are equally efficacious.

Treatment should be given to everyone, even if the chances of giving a second dose are remote, as even a single dose when given even in advanced labor has

Table 4.5 Various tocolytic agents used in preterm labor

Drug	Mechanism of action	Dose	Contraindications	Side effects
Ritodrine	β-adrenergic receptor agonist; reduce intracellular Ca to inhibit myometrial contraction	150 mg in 500 mL solution to be given 300 μg/min	Cardiac diseases, hyperthyroidism, asthma, anemia	Pulmonary edema, acute respiratory distress
Terbutaline	β-agonist		Heart disease, asthma	Pulmonary edema
Magnesium sulfate		4 g loading dose intravenously followed by infusion 2 g/h	Myasthenia gravis, concurrent use of calcium channel blockers	Pulmonary edema, bone loss in fetus if used more than 5 days
Indomethacin	Prostaglandin inhibitor	50–100 mg oral 8 hourly total 200 mg in 24 hours	Renal diseases	Oligohydramnios, intraventricular hemorrhage, premature closure of ductus arteriosus, necrotizing enterocolitis in fetus
Nifedipine	Calcium channel blocker	20 mg followed by 10–20 mg every 8 hourly (maximum 48 hours)	Patients on magnesium sulfate	Reflux tachycardia Decreased atrioventricular conduction
Atosiban	Oxytocin antagonist	6.75 mg over 1 minute loading followed by 6–18 mg/h (maximum 330 mg)		Nausea, headache

Source: World Health Organization recommendation on the use of tocolytic treatment for inhibiting preterm labour. 2015. https://extranet.who.int/rhl/topics/preconception-pregnancy-childbirth-and-postpartum-care/pregnancy-complications/preterm-birth/who-recommendation-use-tocolytic-treatment-inhibiting-preterm-labour.

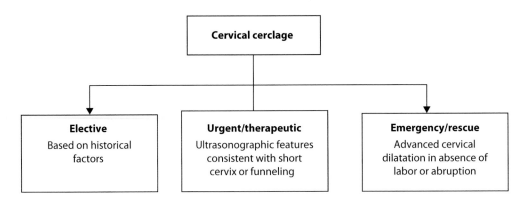

Figure 4.4 Types of cervical cerclage. (From ACOG Practice Bulletin, No. 48, November 2003. Cervical insufficiency. *Int J Gynecol Obstet.* 2004;85[1]:81–9.)

been found to be beneficial. The advantage of corticosteroids is greatest at 2–7 days after the initial dose. A repeat course of corticosteroids should be given if gestation is less than 34 0/7 weeks for those who are at risk of preterm delivery within 7 days, provided more than 14 days have lapsed since the previous course was given. A repeat course may be given as early as 7 days if the clinical scenario indicates. More than two serial courses are not recommended. A rescue dose in cases of PPROM is controversial.

Neonates who have received prenatal corticosteroids have less risk of respiratory distress syndrome, intracranial hemorrhage, necrotizing enterocolitis, and death compared to neonates of same gestational age and weight who have not received corticosteroids.

Role of prenatal magnesium sulfate

Magnesium sulfate is indicated if gestation is less than 32 weeks with imminent preterm birth in the following conditions [18]:

- Women in active labor with cervical dilatation greater than 4 cm with failed tocolysis or tocolytics are contraindicated.
- Cervical os more than 4 cm dilated and progressive dilatation are documented.
- PPROM with active labor.
- Planned delivery for fetal or maternal indication.

It can be used in singleton pregnancy or multifetal gestation, and in both anticipated vaginal or cesarean delivery.

Contraindications:

- Magnesium sulfate is already given for preeclampsia or eclampsia.
- Less than 12 hours have lapsed since discontinuation of previous magnesium sulfate.
- Magnesium sulfate is contraindicated.
- The fetus is not likely to benefit from the therapy.

Dose: Magnesium sulfate is given in a loading dose of 4 g intravenously over 30 minutes, and a maintenance dose of 1 g per hour infusion until delivery or for a maximum of 24 hours. The minimum necessary time of exposure for the fetus is 4 hours prior to delivery.

Monitoring: Maternal blood pressure, respiratory rate, pulse rate, urine output, and patellar reflexes should be checked hourly. Stop the infusion if respiratory rate is less than 12 breaths per minute, patellar reflexes are absent, or urine output falls to less than 100 mL over 4 hours.

Fetal monitoring involves getting a cardiotocograph every 4 hours when the patient is in the latent phase of labor. Continuous electronic fetal monitoring in the active phase of labor is recommended by ACOG.

Strategies with limited or no role in prevention of recurrent preterm birth

Treatment of bacterial vaginosis: Current evidence does not suggest prophylactic treatment of bacterial vaginosis in pregnancy or during the interconception period in patients with a history of spontaneous preterm delivery.

Bed rest: There is no evidence to support bed rest or hospitalization as being effective in the prevention of preterm birth. After 3 days of hospitalization, the risk of venous thromboembolism increases to 1.6% when compared to 0.1% in ambulatory women, along with risk of bone loss.

Smoking cessation and abstaining from the use of illicit substances does have some preventive effect. Prophylactic treatment with broad-spectrum antibiotics for lower genital tract infections and pelvic inflammatory infection does not prevent preterm births. Although gingival infections have been found to be associated with recurrent preterm delivery, treating the same will not prevent them from happening.

CONCLUSION

Recurrent preterm births are associated with not only neonatal morbidity and mortality but also psychological trauma to the woman and caregivers. Establishment of the causative factor is not always possible, as sometimes it can be multifactorial. Serial ultrasound measurements of cervical length to find a short cervix as the cause of preterm birth and applying a cervical stitch where indicated and use of progesterones are some preventive methods. The use of corticosteroids, magnesium sulfate for fetal neuroprotection, and tocolytics in case of established preterm labor to improve perinatal outcome are highly recommended.

REFERENCES

1. Lawn JE, Gravett MG, Nunes TM, Rubens CE, Stanton C. Global report on preterm birth and stillbirth (1 of 7): Definitions, description of the burden and opportunities to improve data. *BMC Pregnancy Childbirth*. 2010;10(S1).
2. Beck S, Wojdyla D, Say L et al. the worldwide incidence of preterm birth: a systematic review of maternal mortality and morbidity. *Bull World Health Organ*. 2010;88(1):31–8.
3. American College of Obstetricians and Gynecologists; Society for Maternal-Fetal Medicine. Obstetric care consensus No. 6: Periviable Birth. *Obstet Gynecol*. 2017;130:e187–99.
4. Nimalkar SM, Bansal SC. Periviable birth: The ethical conundrum. *Indian Pediatr*. 2019;56(1):13–7.
5. Santhakumaran S, Statnikov Y, Gray D on behalf of the Medicines for Neonates Investigator Group, et al. Survival of very preterm infants admitted to neonatal care in England 2008–2014: Time trends and regional variation. *Arch Dis Child Fetal Neonatal Ed*. 2018;103:F208–15.
6. Patel R. Short and long term outcomes for extremely preterm infants. *Am J Perinatol*. 2016;33(03):318–28.
7. López Bernal A. Overview. Preterm labour: Mechanisms and management. *BMC Pregnancy Childbirth*. 2007;7(Suppl 1):S2.
8. Mazaki-Tovi S, Romero R, Kusanovic JP et al. Recurrent preterm birth. *Semin Perinatol*. 2007;31(3):142–58.
9. Bianchi-Jassir F, Seale AC, Kohli-Lynch M et al. Preterm birth associated with group B streptococcus maternal colonization worldwide: Systematic review and meta-analysis. *Clin Infect Dis*. 2017;65(Suppl 2):S133–42.
10. Agrawal V, Hirsch E. Intrauterine infection and preterm labor. *Semin Fetal Neonat Med*. 2012;17(1):12–9.
11. Berghella V. Universal cervical length screening for prediction and prevention of preterm birth. *Obstet Gynecol Surv*. 2012;67(10):653–7.
12. Mercer, B. Preterm premature rupture of membranes. *Obstet Gynecol*. 2003;101(1):178–93.
13. Di Renzo GC, Roura LC, Facchinetti F et al. Guidelines for the management of spontaneous preterm labor: Identification of spontaneous preterm labor, diagnosis of preterm premature rupture of membranes, and preventive tools for preterm birth. *J Matern Fetal Neonatal Med*. 2011;24(5):659–67.
14. ACOG Practice Bulletin, No. 48, November 2003. Cervical insufficiency. *Int J Gynecol Obstet*. 2004;85(1):81–9.
15. Owen J, Hankins G, Iams JD et al. Multicentre randomized trial of cerclage for preterm birth prevention in high-risk women with shortened midtrimester cervical length. *Am J Obstet Gynecol*. 2009;201:375.e1–8.
16. Wise J. NICE guidelines aims to cut premature birth rates. *BMJ*. 2015;351:h6253.

17. Committee Opinion No. 713. *Obstet Gynecol.* 2017;130(2):e102–9.
18. Committee Opinion No. 455. Magnesium sulfate before anticipated preterm birth for neuroprotection. *Obstet Gynecol.* 2010;115(3):669–71.
19. World Health Organization recommendation on the use of tocolytic treatment for inhibiting preterm labour. 2015 https://extranet.who.int/rhl/topics/preconception-pregnancy-childbirth-and-postpartum-care/pregnancy-complications/preterm-birth/who-recommendation-use-tocolytic-treatment-inhibiting-preterm-labour.
20. Jin X, Li D, Huang L. Cervical pessary for prevention of preterm birth: A meta-analysis. *Sci Rep.* 2017;7(1).
21. Wise J. NICE guideline aims to cut premature birth rates. *BMJ.* 2015;351:h6253–h6253.

5

Approach to women with a history of previous intrauterine growth restriction

MINAKSHI ROHILLA

INTRODUCTION

Intrauterine growth restriction (IUGR) is the term applied to a fetus when estimated fetal weight is less than the 10th percentile for that period of gestation or abdominal circumference on ultrasound is less than the 10th percentile [1]. This definition does not include fetuses that are small for gestational age (SGA) but are not pathologically small. However, approximately 50%–70% of fetuses are constitutionally small, and their weight is appropriate for their maternal height, weight, parity, and ethnicity and may be appropriately termed as SGA without any etiologically relevant growth restriction [2]. True growth restriction is a pathologic entity wherein a fetus fails to achieve its expected growth potential irrespective of its genetic constitution. IUGR may be symmetric or asymmetric, depending on the ratio of head circumference to abdominal circumference (HC/AC) (Figure 5.1).

Asymmetric IUGR usually results because of delayed insult to the fetus (e.g., placental insufficiency); hence, the cell size is affected and not the cell number. Such fetuses show a brain-sparing effect and have normal growth of brain and head and hence a higher HC/AC ratio. The fetus redistributes blood flow to sustain function and growth of vital organs; this is called the *brain-sparing effect* and results in increased blood flow to the brain, heart, adrenals, and placenta, with decreased flow to other organs. These different fetal development patterns hence result in IUGR. Symmetric IUGR develops secondary to genetic diseases, but fetal aneuploidy or fetal infection during early fetal life may lead to a uniformly small fetus with a normal HC/AC ratio on ultrasonography. Symmetric IUGR is less common than asymmetric IUGR, and the prognosis for the fetus is mostly guarded, related to the etiology. Prenatal serial fetal growth monitoring and surveillance are less likely to revert the prognosis if IUGR is secondarily due to early fetal insult. Constitutional small or nonpathologic SGA fetuses are also uniformly small (Table 5.1). It is important to distinguish between constitutionally (physiologically) small versus pathologic IUGR fetuses so that maternal and fetal morbidity in view of premature delivery can be avoided in a nonpathologic SGA fetus. It is a clinical challenge

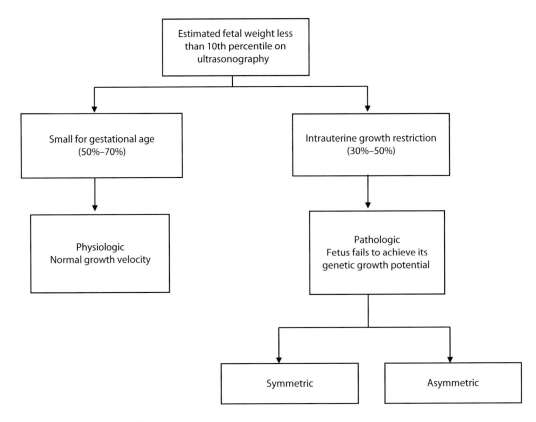

Figure 5.1 Classification of intrauterine growth restriction.

to identify an IUGR fetus with a treatable cause, where timely diagnosis, monitoring of the pregnancy, and exact planning of the delivery will be helpful. The approach to women with a previous history of IUGR requires critical evaluation from the preconceptional period related to the type and cause of IUGR, as well as the possibility of prevention and recurrence of IUGR, accordingly.

Table 5.1 Types of intrauterine growth restriction (IUGR)

Symmetric IUGR	Asymmetric IUGR
Fetus is uniformly small	Head of the fetus is larger than its abdomen
Normal head circumference (HC)/ abdominal circumference (AC)	HC/AC ratio is increased
Etiology: genetic diseases or fetal infection	Chronic placental insufficiency
Poor prognosis	Good prognosis
Included constitutionally small babies	

ETIOLOGY

Various etiological factors have been proposed and found associated with IUGR. Chronic maternal conditions, fetal abnormalities, and abnormal placentation have been implicated in the pathogenesis of IUGR [3]. Any chronic disease with maternal and/or placental vascular involvement leading to decreased placental exchange may cause IUGR. Environmental exposure to toxins including excessive smoking and drug abuse with decreased oxygen-carrying capacity of the mother are rare causes of IUGR (Table 5.2).

SCREENING

Screening involves careful assessment of pregnancies with the potential risk of fetal growth restriction. Critical review of personal, medical, and obstetric history to screen for risk factors that have predictive effects on the outcome of the present pregnancy is required [4]. Screening also involves a decreased value of biochemical parameters like PAPP-A (plasma-associated placental protein–A, less than 0.04 multiple of median) in the current pregnancy to further judge for the possibility of the occurrence of IUGR. PAPP-A is one of the markers of dual screening done routinely to assess the risk of aneuploidy during early pregnancy. IUGR in a previous pregnancy is one of the major risk factors in the present pregnancy for further evaluation (Tables 5.3 and 5.4). Correct assessment of gestational age is the foremost thing to do before diagnosis and detailed evaluation of IUGR. A woman presenting with a history of a previous SGA neonate needs a detailed obstetric history to assess for the type and cause of IUGR of that pregnancy. All prenatal records and delivery details should be reviewed to know the possible etiology of IUGR. A critical appraisal regarding the birth weight, morphology, obvious congenital malformation, and subsequent gain in the weight of the newborn is required. Maternal evaluation for past or present hypertension, diabetes mellitus, substance abuse, antiphospholipid antibody syndrome, poor dietary habits, and chronic infections like tuberculosis, syphilis, and malaria are required prepregnancy. A woman with a history of chronic hypertension or preeclampsia should be administered tablet aspirin for prevention of recurrence of preeclampsia and subsequent IUGR. A pregnant woman with a history of IUGR has a high risk of recurrence of IUGR (odds ratio greater than 2) and hence will require serial fetal growth monitoring and umbilical artery Doppler studies from 26 to 28 weeks' gestation as a method of screening for IUGR in the current pregnancy.

Table 5.2 Etiological factors of intrauterine growth restriction

Maternal	Fetal	Placental
Hypertensive disorders	Chromosomal abnormalities	Abruption
Pregestational diabetes	Structural malformations	Infarction
Renal diseases	Multiple gestation	Circumvallate
Autoimmune diseases		Hemangioma
Multiple gestation		Chorioangioma
Exposure to teratogens		Abnormal cord insertion
Antophospholipid antibody		Single umbilical artery
Substance abuse		
Infectious diseases		

Source: American College of Obstetricians and Gynecologists. *Obstet Gynecol.* 2013;121:1122–33.

Table 5.3 History of risk factors in present or past pregnancy

Major risk factors (Odds ratio >2)	Minor risk factors (Odds ratio 1–2)
Maternal age more than 40 years	Maternal age more than 35 years
Smoker more than 11 cigarettes/day	Nulliparity
Cocaine abuse	Smoker less than 10 cigarettes/day
Previous baby with intrauterine growth restriction	*In vitro* fertilization pregnancy
History of stillbirth	Prepregnancy fruit intake was low
Maternal/paternal small for gestational age	History of preeclampsia
Chronic hypertension	Pregnancy interval less than 6 months or more
Diabetes with vasculopathy	than 60 months
Chronic kidney disease	
Antiphospholipid syndrome	

Source: Royal College of Obstetricians and Gynecologists. *The Investigation and Management of the Small for Gestational Age Fetus. Green-top Guideline No. 31,* 2nd ed. London, UK: Royal College of Obstetricians and Gynecologists; 2013.

Table 5.4 Risk factors in current pregnancy

Major risk factors (Odds ratio >2)	Minor risk factors (Odds ratio 1–2)
Threatened miscarriage	Mild preeclampsia
Fetal anomaly scan showing echogenic bowel	Placental abruption
Preeclampsia	Caffeine intake greater than
Pregnancy-induced hypertension with severe features	300 mg/day in third
Prepartum hemorrhage (unexplained)	trimester
Inadequate maternal weight gain	
Maternal infections (e.g., tuberculosis, syphilis, malaria, etc.)	
Plasma-associated placental protein–A less than 0.4 multiple of medians	

Source: Royal College of Obstetricians and Gynecologists. *The Investigation and Management of the Small for Gestational Age Fetus. Green-top Guideline No. 31,* 2nd ed. London, UK: Royal College of Obstetricians and Gynecologists; 2013.

Measurement of uterine fundal height/symphysis fundal height

Measurement of symphysis fundal height (SFH)/ uterine fundal height is an excellent screening tool for assessment of IUGR after 24–26 weeks of gestation. Discrepancy of more than 3 cm is indicative of probable growth restriction and calls for further evaluation [5]. In women with body mass index greater than 35, large fibroids, hydramnios, and multiple gestation, SFH measurement alone is inaccurate, and serial assessment of fetal size using ultrasound is recommended.

Role of uterine artery Doppler in screening of intrauterine growth restriction

Uterine artery Doppler is recommended if more than three minor risk factors for IUGR are present (Figure 5.2) [4]. With the advancement of gestational age, uterine artery diastolic flow falls due to invasion of spiral arteries by trophoblast cells. This results in loss of diastolic notch by 18–22 weeks of gestation. A pulsatility index (PI) greater than the 95th percentile or notch in uterine artery Doppler is suggestive of uteroplacental insufficiency (Figure 5.3a through c).

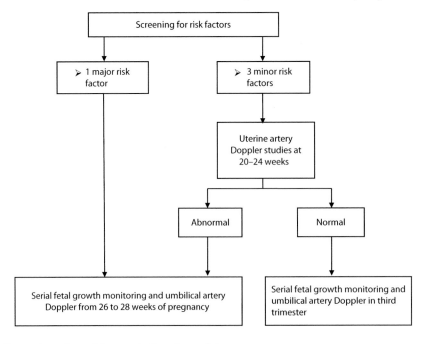

Figure 5.2 Screening of small for gestational age fetuses.

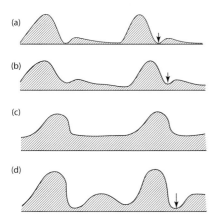

Figure 5.3 Doppler waveform of uterine artery blood flow: (a) Normal in first trimester, (b) normal in early second and third trimesters, (c) normal in third trimester, and (d) in preeclampsia after 24 weeks of gestation.

Abnormal flow warrants umbilical artery Doppler studies at 26–28 weeks of gestation onward. There is no role of uterine artery Doppler study in a woman presenting with major risk factors in a current pregnancy, like a previous history of IUGR, but serial growth monitoring and antepartum fetal surveillance are needed once fetal viability is achieved.

INVESTIGATIONS

Investigations recommended in a woman with an IUGR fetus are summarized in Table 5.5. A woman with a history of unexplained IUGR in a previous pregnancy should not miss dual screening for risk of aneuploidy with PAPP-A as a biochemical marker and early scanning for fetal anomaly to rule out intrinsic fetal causes of IUGR in the present

Table 5.5 Investigations

Detailed fetal anatomic survey at 18–20 weeks
Karyotyping in fetuses with severe intrauterine growth restriction, especially when uterine artery Doppler and amniotic fluid are normal
Screening for cytomegalovirus, toxoplasmosis by serological examination
Testing for malaria and syphilis in a population who is at high risk for these infections

Source: Royal College of Obstetricians and Gynecologists. *The Investigation and Management of the Small for Gestational Age Fetus. Green-top Guideline No. 31*, 2nd ed. London, UK: Royal College of Obstetricians and Gynecologists; 2013.

pregnancy. Detailed anatomical survey by level II obstetric ultrasonography, fetal echocardiography, karyotyping in case of fetal structural anomaly, and serological screening for congenital cytomegalovirus, toxoplasmosis, syphilis, and malaria infection should be offered, especially if there is an early-onset severe IUGR. The rate of aneuploidy may be as high as 20% in the case of early-onset severe IUGR independent of a structurally anomalous fetus [4]. All other investigations according to the maternal morbidity and associated factors of IUGR need to be done. For example, a woman with a chronic medical illness with IUGR should also have serial workups of investigations related to the progression or stability of the disease and to know the further course or prognosis of IUGR.

DIAGNOSIS OF FETAL GROWTH RESTRICTION

Sonographic measurement of fetal size

Objective fetal growth estimation using various fetal biometric measurements is recommended from 26 weeks of gestation onward. This includes combined head, abdomen, and femur bone measurements to estimate fetal growth velocity and prediction of growth restriction using customized fetal weight reference charts. Customized charts are specific for race, ethnicity, height, weight, and parity. Fetuses with weight less than the third percentile of reference have severe growth restriction, which is associated with poor obstetrical outcomes. However, in a low-risk population, perinatal outcome does not improve with the use of routine fetal biometry.

Amniotic fluid volume measurement

Approximately 10% of pregnancies with oligohydramnios are associated with fetal growth restriction [6], probably due to chronic hypoxia and reduced fetal renal perfusion. Measurement of amniotic fluid index is must in cases of suspected growth restriction, oligohydramnious further supports the diagnosis of IUGR [7]. Estimation of a single deepest vertical pocket (SDVP) of more than 2 cm has been found to be more specific than measurement of amniotic fluid index (AFI). As per recent literature, more cases of oligohydramnios were diagnosed and more women had induction of labor with AFI $\geq$ 5 cm than SDVP; however, there was no improvement in perinatal outcome [4].

MANAGEMENT OF GROWTH-RESTRICTED FETUSES

Role of cardiotocography

Fetal heart variation is the most useful parameter of cardiotocography (CTG) for prediction of well-being of IUGR fetuses. Short-term variability of less than 3 ms should be considered as a consistent marker of fetal acidemia, and delivery should be planned within 24 hours [8]. Computerized CTG (cCTG) is more objective and specific and has less inter- and intraobserver variation than conventional CTG [9].

Biophysical profile

The biophysical profile (BPP) includes five fetal parameters: fetal breathing movement, fetal tone, body movement, amniotic fluid index and cardiotocography, each assigned a score of two, making a total score of 10/10 in a normal fetus. A normal biophysical profile has a very low false-negative rate (0%) and perinatal mortality within 7 days of testing (0.2%). However, in extremely premature and severe IUGR (<1 kg), BPP has a high false-negative rate (11%) and has not been recommended for fetal surveillance [4].

Role of Doppler studies

Doppler study is used along with nonstress tests and biophysical profiles in the management of growth-restricted fetuses. Doppler study of various fetal vessels like umbilical artery and umbilical vein, middle cerebral artery, and ductus venosus (DV) can predict perinatal morbidity and mortality in IUGR fetuses associated with absent or reversed end diastolic flow (AREDF) and aids in decision making regarding the timing of termination of pregnancy.

S/D ratio: Systolic/diastolic ratio
(S-D)/S: Resistance index (RI)
(S-D)/Mean: Pulsatility index (PI)

Umbilical artery Doppler

Umbilical artery Doppler should be the primary surveillance tool in IUGR fetuses. An umbilical artery Doppler is recommended after 24 weeks of pregnancy in case of a high risk of IUGR in the current pregnancy or with abnormal uterine artery

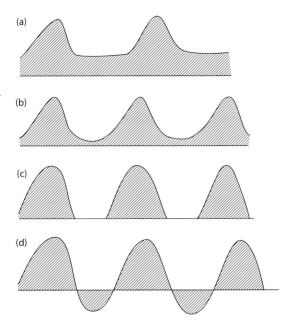

Figure 5.4 Doppler study of umbilical artery blood flow: (a) Normal Doppler flow velocity, (b) high pulsatility index, (c) absent end diastolic flow, and (d) reversed end diastolic flow.

Doppler studies during screening in a woman with minor risk factors [4,7]. The normal mean value of the umbilical artery S/D ratio (systolic/diastolic ratio) decreases from 3.6 to 2.5 as the gestation advances (Figure 5.4a). IUGR fetuses with placental insufficiency may have an increased pulsatility index (PI) (i.e., PI more than two standard deviations (Figure 5.4b) for gestational age in the umbilical artery), which may subsequently worsen to absent end diastolic flow (AEDF) (Figure 5.4c) and reversed end diastolic flow (REDF) (Figure 5.4d). In comparison to CTG, umbilical artery Doppler is associated with a smaller number of inductions of labor and cesarean sections for fetal distress [10].

Fetal middle cerebral artery Doppler

The physiologic basis behind Doppler changes in the middle cerebral artery (MCA) is that in cases of placental insufficiency, blood supply to essential organs like the brain is maintained, which is also known as the "brain-sparing effect." It has importance in the assessment of fetal cardiovascular status, fetal anemia, and fetal hypoxia. A PI less than the fifth percentile suggests fetal acidosis in an IUGR fetus. MCA Doppler is useful to predict the timing of delivery when IUGR is diagnosed after

32 weeks' gestation, especially when umbilical artery Doppler is normal. In a prospective study of 210 term fetuses with normal umbilical artery Doppler, the PI of a MCA Doppler study less than the fifth percentile was predictive of fetal distress and neonatal acidosis, which was confirmed with low umbilical artery pH and base deficit in the newborn [11].

Ductus venosus and umbilical vein Doppler

DV Doppler should be used in the surveillance of IUGR fetuses, which have abnormal umbilical artery Doppler. This surveillance is important in deciding the timing of delivery. A normal waveform of DV includes three peaks of ventricular systole, early diastole, and atrial contraction, respectively (Figure 5.5a). The absence of a wave (Figure 5.5b) or reversal of a wave in DV (Figure 5.5c) suggests fetal hypoxia, and delivery is recommended. Pulsatility in the umbilical vein suggests fetal cardiac compromise, and urgent delivery is suggested.

In IUGR fetuses with normal umbilical artery Doppler, fetal surveillance at 2-week intervals is reasonable, while in the case of an abnormal umbilical artery PI, twice weekly and daily surveillance in AREDF is mandatory [4].

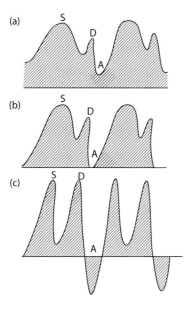

Figure 5.5 Doppler flow velocity of ductus venosus: (a) Normal, (b) absent A wave, and (c) reversed A wave.

APPROACH TO WOMEN WITH IUGR IN CURRENT AND PAST PREGNANCIES

The management of growth-restricted fetuses (Figures 5.6 and 5.7) depends on confirmation of diagnosis, fetal condition, and associated maternal factors. Screening for IUGR should be initiated during preconceptional counseling or the first prenatal visit and should be reassessed around 20 weeks' gestation. If the cause of IUGR in previous pregnancy seems to be a recurrent chronic medical condition, like hypertension, diabetes, renal disease, and autoimmune diseases, stabilization of the disease is necessary before planning the next pregnancy. Advice on diet and lifestyle modifications should be part of the preconceptional counseling. It is important to reconfirm the period of gestation and exclude a constitutionally small fetus before the diagnosis of SGA fetus is established. It is essential to do fetal aneuploidy screen by dual screen, early fetal anomaly scan with nuchal translucency and presence of nasal bone at 11–13 weeks' gestation, and level II ultrasonography and fetal CTG to exclude obvious structural malformations. Apart from surveillance of an IUGR fetus, maternal evaluation for any associated comorbidities like preeclampsia and chronic hypertension or renal and autoimmune disease, and management of that particular disease, are also required in the current pregnancy. A woman presenting with a previous history of IUGR requires fetal growth monitoring at 2- to 3-week intervals along with a biophysical profile and umbilical artery Doppler as a screening method to detect IUGR, once fetal viability is achieved. Once IUGR is established in the current pregnancy, there are many methods available for prepartum fetal surveillance, and all aim to envisage fetal acidosis prior to multiorgan dysfunction of the fetus and fetal death. These are biophysical profile, fetal CTG, and Doppler study of the umbilical artery, middle cerebral artery, umbilical vein, and ductus venosus. If umbilical artery Doppler study is normal with evidence of some serial fetal growth and the biophysical profile is satisfactory, then pregnancy may be continued until 37–38 weeks' gestation with 2- to 3-week fetal biometry and weekly biophysical profiles. If the PI of the umbilical artery Doppler study is high, a biweekly biophysical profile should continue with MCA Doppler study starting at 32 weeks' gestation. If MCA Doppler

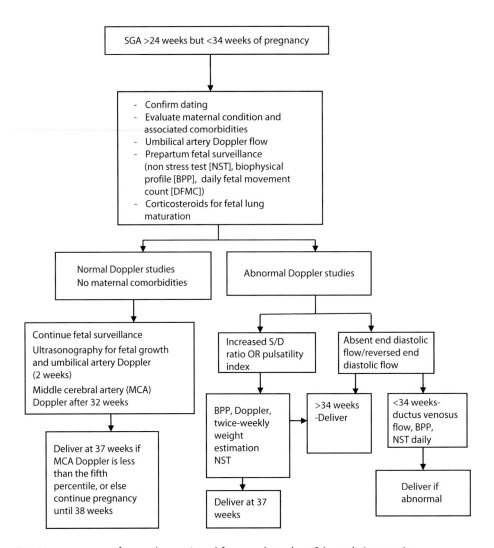

Figure 5.6 Management of growth-restricted fetus at less than 34 weeks' gestation.

study along with BPP is normal, pregnancy may be continued until 37–38 weeks' gestation. Delivery is recommended at 37 weeks' gestation if the PI of the MCA Doppler is less than the fifth percentile or fetal growth is static for 3 weeks at any time after 34 weeks' gestation. Pregnancy needs to be terminated at 32–34 weeks' gestation in the case of AEDF/REDF in Doppler study of the umbilical artery. If AEDF/REDF occurs before 32–34 weeks' gestation, daily biophysical profile along with Doppler study of DV needs to be added to decide timing of delivery. The absence of a wave or reversal of a wave in DV predicts fetal acidosis, and delivery is recommended. Steroids for fetal lung maturity should be given to the mother if delivery is planned at or before 34 weeks' gestation or if elective cesarean

section is contemplated before 39 weeks' gestation [4,12]. Maternal administration of magnesium sulfate is also recommended for neuroprotection and to reduce the incidence of cerebral palsy in the newborn, in case of planned delivery before 32 weeks' gestation.

MODE OF DELIVERY

In IUGR fetuses with umbilical artery AREDF, cesarean section is recommended. However, in fetuses with abnormal umbilical artery Doppler, induction of labor may be offered with an anticipated high risk of emergency cesarean section. Continuous fetal CTG is recommended as soon as uterine contractions begin. Computerized

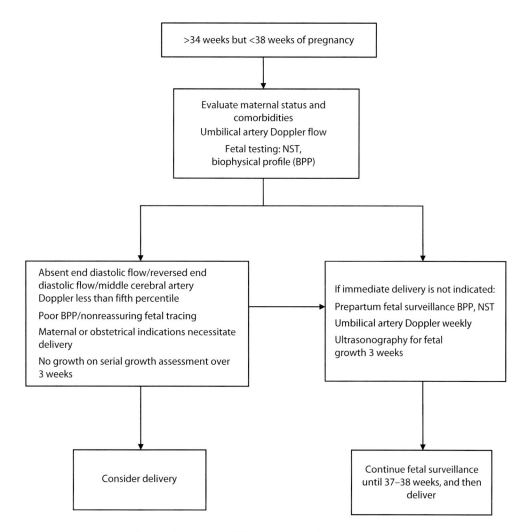

Figure 5.7 Management of growth-restricted fetus at more than 34 weeks' gestation.

interpretation of the CTG based on short-term variability is a better predictor of fetal compromise or ongoing hypoxia [4].

COMPLICATIONS ASSOCIATED WITH IUGR

Various complications (Table 5.6) have been found to be associated with IUGR fetuses along with a higher association of diabetes and atherosclerosis in later life due to metabolic derangements of IUGR in the past, known as the "Barker hypothesis" [13].

PREVENTION

Prevention of growth restriction is possible if modifiable risk factors like optimization of maternal health and nutrition, avoiding drugs causing IUGR, cessation of smoking, and decreasing caffeine intake are identified and appropriate measures are preferably taken before conception. Low-dose aspirin is recommended for prophylaxis of IUGR before 16 weeks of gestation if a woman is at high risk for preeclampsia [4]. The use of multivitamins, calcium supplements, progesterone, bed rest, or dietary modifications is not recommended.

IUGR is an important obstetric condition that is best prevented. A careful screening of at-risk pregnancies, an early objective diagnosis, and diligent monitoring is the cornerstone of its management. In the majority of cases, the etiology remains obscure and warrants vigilant surveillance. Early supervision and careful monitoring of pregnancy along with well-timed delivery can reduce perinatal

Table 5.6 Complications associated with intrauterine growth restriction

Fetal	Neonatal	Adult
Increased rate of stillbirth	Meconium aspiration syndrome	Risk of hypertension
Birth asphyxia	Neonatal hypoglycemia	Type 2 diabetes mellitus
Prematurity	Hypothermia	Atherosclerosis
	Hyperbilirubinemia	
	Intraventricular hemorrhage	
	Necrotizing enterocolitis	
	Seizures	
	Sepsis	
	Respiratory distress	
	Syndrome	
	Neonatal death	

Source: McIntire DD et al. *N Engl J Med.* 1999;340:1234–8; McIntire DD et al. *N Engl J Med.* 1999;340:1234–8.

morbidity and mortality. Judicious use of modern techniques of fetal and maternal Doppler studies, BPP, and computed CTG have changed the outlook of management of IUGR.

REFERENCES

1. Chang TC, Robson SC, Boys RJ, Spencer JA. Prediction of the small for gestational age infant: Which ultrasonic measurement is best? *Obstet Gynecol.* 1992;80:1030–8.
2. Alberry M, Soothill P. Management of fetal growth restriction. *Arch Dic Child Fetal Neonatal Ed.* 2007;92:62–7.
3. American College of Obstetricians and Gynecologists. ACOG Practice bulletin no. 134: Fetal growth restriction. *Obstet Gynecol.* 2013;121:1122–33.
4. Royal College of Obstetricians and Gynecologists. *The Investigation and Management of the Small for Gestational Age Fetus. Green-top Guideline No. 31*, 2nd ed. London, UK: Royal College of Obstetricians and Gynecologists; 2013.
5. Figueras F, Gardosi J. Intrauterine growth restriction: New concepts in antenatal surveillance, diagnosis, and management. *Am J Obstet Gynecol.* 2011;204(4):288.
6. Chauhan SP, Taylor M, Sheilds D et al. Intrauterine growth restriction and oligohydramnios among high risk patients. *Am J Perinatol.* 2007;24(4):215.
7. Lausman A, Kingdom J; Maternal Fetal Medicine Committee. Intrauterine growth restriction: Screening, diagnosis and management. *J Obstet Gynaecol Can.* 2013;35(8):741–57.
8. Serra V, Moulden M, Bellver J, Redman CW. The value of the short-term fetal heart rate variation for timing the delivery of the growth–retarded fetuses. *BJOG.* 2008;115:1101–7.
9. Serra V, Bellver J, Moulden M, Redman CW. Computerized analysis of normal fetal heart rate pattern throughout gestation. *Ultrasound Obstet Gynecol.* 2009;34:74–9.
10. Williams KP, Farquharson DF, Bebbington M et al. Screening for fetal wellbeing in a high risk pregnant population comparing the nonstress test with umbilical artery Doppler velocimetry: A randomized controlled clinical trial. *Am J Obstet Gynecol.* 2003;188:1366–71.
11. Cruz–Martinez R, Figueras F, Hernandez–Andrade E, Oros D, Gratecos E. Fetal brain Doppler to predict cesarean delivery for nonreassuring fetal status in term small-for-gestational-age fetuses. *Obstet Gynecol.* 2011;117:618–26.
12. Fetal growth disorders. Cunningham FG, Leveno KJ, Bloom SL et al. editors. *Williams Obstetrics.* 24th ed. New York, NY: McGraw-Hill; 2013. http://accessmedicine.mhmedical.com/content.aspx?bookid=1057&sectionid=59789188.
13. McIntire DD, Bloom SL, Casey BM, Leveno KJ. Birth weight in relation to morbidity and mortality among newborn infants. *N Engl J Med.* 1999;340:1234–8.

6

Protocol for management of late second-trimester and term fetal death

ARUNA SINGH AND PRADIP KUMAR SAHA

INTRODUCTION

Stillbirth is defined as the death of the fetus before the complete expulsion from the mother's womb. There is a lack of uniform consensus regarding the definition of *stillbirth* in terms of different cutoffs for gestational age and fetal weight.

The World Health Organization (WHO) has defined *fetal death* as any death that has occurred irrespective of duration of pregnancy and before complete expulsion from the mother. For international comparison, the WHO has recommended *stillbirth* be defined as a baby born with no signs of life at 28 weeks or more or at a weight of 1000 g or more [1].

The American College of Obstetricians and Gynecologists (ACOG) defines stillbirth as delivery of a fetus that shows no signs of life, e.g., absence of breathing, heartbeat, and pulsations in the umbilical cord. The suggested requirement is to report fetal deaths at 20 weeks or greater of gestation (if the gestational age is known) or a weight greater than or equal to 350 g if the gestational age is not known. The cutoff of 350 g is the 50th percentile for weight at 20 weeks' gestation [2].

The *Perinatal Mortality Surveillance Report* (CEMACH) adapted by the Royal College of Obstetricians and Gynaecologists (RCOG) defines *stillbirth* as "a baby delivered with no signs of life known to have died after 24 completed weeks of pregnancy." *Intrauterine fetal death* (IUFD) refers to babies with no signs of life *in utero* [3].

In India, the Ministry of Health and Family Welfare (MOHFW) has defined late fetal death as death of a fetus weighing at least 1000 g (or a gestational age of 28 completed weeks or a crown-heel length of 35 cm or more) [4].

There is no single definition of stillbirth. Various definitions have been suggested by different bodies over the years based on the feasibility of neonatal care and individual country perspective (Table 6.1).

Terminology regarding stillbirth is complicated and confusing due to the following [5]:

- Discrepancy regarding birth weight versus gestational age
- Interpretation problems when there is discrepancy between the gestational age of fetal demise and at delivery

Table 6.1 Definitions of stillbirth

Definition suggested by	Gestational age cutoff	Birth weight cutoff	Fetal length	Remarks
Royal College of Obstetricians and Gynaecologists (RCOG)	≥24 weeks			
World Health Organization	≥28 weeks	≥1000 grams	≥35 cm	
Centers for Disease Control and Prevention	Early 20–27 weeks Late 28–36 weeks Term >37 weeks			
India (MOHFW, 2016)	Early 20–28 weeks Late ≥28 weeks	500 grams 1000 grams	≥25 cm ≥35 cm	
American College of Obstetricians and Gynecologists (ACOG)	≥20 weeks	≥350 grams	—	350 g is the 50th percentile for weight at 20 weeks' gestation

- Incomplete data from low-income countries where many births occur at home and in remote areas

Stillbirth is defined as loss after 20 weeks period of gestation (POG) (early stillbirth [20–27 weeks], late stillbirth [28–36 weeks], and term stillbirth [greater than 37 weeks]) by the U.S. National Center for Health Statistics [6]. Uncomplicated pregnancy shows almost half of these, with most occurring prior to the onset of labor [7].

When comparing stillbirth rates globally, the rates of late stillbirths are used (those 28 weeks of gestation or later). Approximately 98% of these stillbirths occur in low-income countries. Rates of stillbirth in low-income countries have been substantially higher (approximately 21 deaths/1000 live births) than in high-income countries (approximately 3 deaths/1000 live births). However, declines in the past decade have been reported. A study in low- and middle-income countries found a 3% decline in stillbirth from 2010 to 2016 [8].

ETIOLOGY AND RISK FACTORS FOR STILLBIRTH

Maternal causes

Diabetes: Women with diabetes are at increased risk of sudden fetal demise at term. A study from the United States reported that the term stillbirth rate among women with diabetes is more than twice as high as the rate in the overall obstetric population [9]. Hyperglycemia is one cause of stillbirth in diabetic pregnancies, but fetal congenital anomalies, heart defects, intrauterine growth restriction (IUGR), and vasculopathy are additional risk factors.

Hypertensive disorders: Hypertensive disorders are a leading cause of stillbirths, particularly in low-income countries. Placental insufficiency and abruption are the major causes of fetal death in women with hypertension.

Intrahepatic cholestasis of pregnancy: Intrahepatic cholestasis of pregnancy (ICP) usually occurs in late pregnancy and causes stillbirth in less than 5% of cases.

Intrauterine growth restriction (IUGR): IUGR is associated with an increased risk of stillbirth, particularly in cases having weight less than 2.5 percentile. The cumulative risk of stillbirth for weight less than the 10th percentile is approximately 1.5% and increases with lower weight [10].

Abruptio placentae: Abruptio placentae accounts for approximately 10%–20% of all stillbirth cases [11]. The risk is highest with central abruption or when more than half of the placental surface is separated. Stillbirth is more commonly seen when abruption occurs in a preterm.

Fetomaternal hemorrhage: Fetal anemia secondary to fetomaternal hemorrhage may cause stillbirth.

Smoking, illicit drugs: Meta-analysis has found that any active maternal smoking was associated with increased risks of stillbirth [12].

Uterine abnormalities: Structural uterine abnormalities, such as a unicornuate uterus, can cause previable preterm birth that can be due to associated cervical insufficiency. A pregnancy in a rudimentary horn may not reach viability.

Platelet alloimmunization: Severe fetal alloimmune thrombocytopenia can result in fetal death *in utero* due to intracranial hemorrhage.

Unexplained

This category constitutes fetal demise that cannot be attributed to any cause with all information available accounting for 25%–60% of all stillbirths. These cases include stillbirths reported as unexplained (or unknown or unclassified), generally reflecting whether stillbirth was fully evaluated, whether the classification system used to assign stillbirth includes risk factors as cause or not. A systematic review of classification systems for stillbirths found that the percentage where the cause of death was unexplained ranged from 0.39% (Nordic-Baltic classification) to 46% (Keeling system) [13].

Fetal causes

Infections: It is estimated that about 19% of stillbirths at less than 28 weeks' gestation and 2% of term stillbirths are attributed to infections. Pathogens commonly causing stillbirths include parvovirus, cytomegalovirus (CMV), syphilis, and *Listeria monocytogenes*. For example, in developing countries, malaria is a cause of stillbirth. Infection accounts for approximately half of infective causes of stillbirths and 10%–25% of stillbirths in high-income countries [7]. Infection may contribute to stillbirth by affecting fetal, maternal, or placental compartment.

In high-income countries, the majority of infection-related stillbirths occur following premature rupture of membranes in periviable fetuses. Lower genital tract infection with ascending spread is the usual mechanism of infection. The rate of these losses has been relatively stable over the past 30 years. Viral, pyogenic, fungal, protozoa and spirochetes are all potential pathogens that can cause transplacental infections with viral as the most common causing hematogenous infection of the placenta. Almost any maternal systemic illness can infect placenta but usually does not lead to fetal demise. CMV and parvovirus infection are the most common to consider among viruses [14].

Due to the relatively high frequency of asymptomatic maternal vaginal carriage and lack of proper diagnostic criterion, there are challenges in assigning infection as a cause of stillbirth, and a histologic confirmation should be attained prior to attributing infection as the causative factor. However, an infected fetus may be unable to mount an immune response at times, so one may not find any evidence of fetal infection.

Genetic/congenital anomalies: Abnormal karyotype is found in approximately 8%–13% of stillbirths and in an even higher percentage in fetuses with anatomical abnormalities. Abdominal wall and neural tube defects, thanatophoric dysplasia, amniotic band, and so on, are associated with risk of stillbirth.

In a study of registry data [15], the isolated anomalies with the highest rates of stillbirth after exclusion of pregnancy terminations were anencephaly (51%), encephalocele (15%), arhinencephaly/holoprosencephaly (12%), hydrocephaly (9%), hypoplastic left or right heart (9%), single cardiac ventricle (9%), spina bifida (6%), gastroschisis or omphalocele (6%), common arterial truncus (4%), and diaphragmatic hernia (3%).

Umbilical cord events: Umbilical cord events like nuchal cord, knots, or other abnormalities accounted for 10% of fetal deaths in one population-based study. Although cord abnormalities are common (occurring in 15%–34% of pregnancies at term) [16], they are rarely severe enough to cause fetal demise.

PREDICTING AT-RISK PREGNANCIES

- Racial factors
- Maternal medical disorders
- Nulliparity
- Cigarette smoking
- Obesity
- Advanced maternal age
- Multiple pregnancy
- Previous stillbirth
- Previous small for gestational age newborn or abruption
- Social issues (unmarried, history of intimate partner violence)
- Recreational use of drugs
- Conception via assisted reproductive technology
- Maternal sleep-disordered breathing

DIAGNOSIS

Ultrasonography is an important tool for the accurate diagnosis of stillbirth.

INVESTIGATIONS TO EVALUATE LATE INTRAUTERINE FETAL DEATH

Aim of investigations

- Assess maternal well-being
- Determine cause of stillbirth
- Determine risk of recurrence and assess preventive measures
- Provide adequate counseling to the parents regarding etiological factors

Tests recommended for women with late IUFD

- *Standard hematology and biochemistry*: For preeclampsia and its complications, to look for evidence of multiple organ dysfunction syndrome (MODS) in sepsis or hemorrhage, platelet testing twice a week for occult disseminated intravascular coagulation (DIC).
- *Coagulation profile and plasma fibrinogen*: Test of maternal well-being; sepsis, preeclampsia, and placental abruption increase chances of DIC.
- Maternal glucose and HbA1c.
- Thyroid function tests.
- *Kleihauer-Betke test*: Fetomaternal hemorrhage is a cause of stillbirth. This test should be undertaken before birth and should be recommended in all women.
- *Bile salts*: For obstetric cholestasis.
- *Tests under special circumstances:*
  - Maternal viral screen, syphilis, tropical infections
  - Maternal thrombophilia screen
  - Parental blood for karyotype
  - Fetal and placental tissue for karyotype/microbiology
- *Role of chromosomal microarray (CMA)*: It is useful in the evaluation of stillbirth. Chromosomal abnormalities are identified in approximately 5% of stillborn fetuses in the absence of an anatomical malformation, and this number increases further to 35%–40% in the presence of structural abnormalities. In these cases, CMA can overcome this difficulty. In cases with

stillbirth, CMA is a preferred option for further evaluation of fetuses with structural abnormalities, after fetal demise (particularly when chromosomal analysis is desired but G-banding is not possible due to failure of cell culture). Some clinicians have advocated a microarray as a first-line test whenever fetal chromosomal analysis is planned.

DELIVERY ISSUES

Timing of delivery

Parents should be given time to fully accept the death of their baby, and they should not be rushed into making any decisions about delivery during this chaotic period in the absence of serious medical concerns in the mother.

Expectant management

Women who are otherwise candidates for vaginal delivery and are medically uncomplicated should be given the option of waiting for spontaneous onset of labor and should be told that spontaneous labor begins in the majority of cases within 1–2 weeks after fetal death. Most women with intrauterine fetal demise have a spontaneous labor within 3 weeks of diagnosis. Testing for DIC should be considered twice weekly. There is a 10% chance of having a DIC within a month from the date of fetal death [17].

Immediate delivery

Sepsis, preeclampsia, placental abruption, ruptured membranes, or DIC necessitate immediate delivery.

MODE OF DELIVERY

- *Vaginal birth*: Recommended for most women
- Cesarean birth required only for maternal indications

Method of induction for unscarred uterus

Mifepristone and a prostaglandin preparation are recommended for the induction of labor [18]. Misoprostol can be used in preference to dinoprost. Only misoprostol or oxytocin can be used as alternatives. Mechanical methods are not recommended.

18–26 WEEKS POG

PGE1, misoprostol can be administered 100 mcg every 6–12 hours for a maximum of four doses in 24 hours. If the first dose does not cause effective contractions, one can double the subsequent dose, total daily dose should not exceed 800 mcg.

OVER 26 WEEKS POG

- Decision is based on cervical findings
- For *favorable cervix*, either misoprostol or oxytocin can be used
- For *unfavorable cervix*, misoprostol, vaginal 25–50 mcg 4 hours apart, up to six doses can be given

If the first dose does not cause effective contractions, the subsequent dose may be doubled. Maximum daily dose should not exceed 600 mcg. If contractions occur (two contractions in 10 minutes), the dose may need to be repeated and intravenous oxytocin may need to be started after 4 hours of the last misoprostol dose. If contractions diminish, repeat misoprostol may be given.

OTHER APPROACHES FOR MIDTRIMESTER PREGNANCIES (24–28 WEEKS POG)

- Misoprostol only 100–200 mcg vaginally 4 hours apart.
- Mifepristone-misoprostol—mifepristone 200 mg or 600 mg per oral followed by misoprostol 24–48 hours later.

High-dose oxytocin can also be used as an alternative, beginning with 6 milliunits/min, increasing by 6 milliunits/min, every 45 minutes (not exceeding 45 milliunits/min) until effective contractions are achieved.

METHOD OF INDUCTION IN SPECIAL POPULATIONS

Previous cesarean delivery

- Patient should be counseled on risks and benefits of vaginal birth, risk of intrapartum rupture (being higher if induced as compared to spontaneous).
- Decisions regarding safety and benefits should be undertaken by the consultant obstetrician.
- Women with previous vertical or classical cesarean should be informed about increased chances of rupture as compared to previous lower-segment cesarean section (LSCS). These women should be offered cesarean delivery, although vaginal delivery is not absolutely contraindicated with late fetal demise.

Second-trimester fetal demise with one previous LSCS

- Misoprostol <200 mcg every 4 hours vaginally
- Mifepristone can be used alone

Third-trimester fetal demise with one previous LSCS

- *Cervix favorable*: Oxytocin in standard doses
- *Cervix unfavorable*: Either mechanical method followed by oxytocin or misoprostol can be used

Women with previous two LSCSs

- A little higher risk with prostaglandins compared to one LSCS
  - Women with more than previous two LSCS or atypical or unknown scars
- Safety of induction of labor unknown

Placenta previa

- Placenta previa in early pregnancy—can conduct vaginal delivery
- Cesarean delivery is a safer option for women over 24 weeks and all third trimester
- Routine antibiotic prophylaxis—not recommended
- Women with evidence of sepsis—broad-spectrum intravenous antibiotics
- Decision of thromboprophylaxis in patients with DIC should be taken in consultation with hematologist

STRATEGIES FOR PREVENTION OF STILLBIRTH

Basic interventions

A systematic review has provided the following steps to reduce the burden of stillbirth worldwide [7,19]:

- Folic acid supplementation
- Down syndrome screening

- Ultrasound examination
  - For confirmation of gestational age (6–8 weeks)
  - For fetal congenital malformations (18–22 weeks)
  - For assessment of fetal growth, amniotic fluid volume, and periodic interval
- Malaria screening and prevention
- Syphilis screening and prevention
- Early diagnosis and management of hypertensive disorders
- Early diagnosis and management of diabetes
- Early diagnosis and management of IUGR
- Early induction of postterm pregnancy
- Skillful birth attendants
- Emergency obstetric care facilities availability
- Comprehensive emergency obstetric care availability

Antepartum fetal monitoring

Doppler velocimetry is used for monitoring the growth-restricted fetus.

The ACOG recommends the initiation of antepartum fetal testing 1–2 weeks prior to the gestational age of the previous stillbirth and by 32–34 weeks of gestation (Figure 6.1) [20,21].

Monitoring fetal movement

Patients who report decreased fetal movement are at increased risk of having an adverse pregnancy outcome, including stillbirth, and approximately half of stillbirths are preceded by decreased fetal movement.

Timing of delivery

Expert consensus guidelines suggest avoiding scheduled delivery before 39 weeks if the previous stillbirth was unexplained and the current pregnancy is uncomplicated (i.e., reassuring fetal testing, no maternal or fetal complications such as preeclampsia or growth restriction, no maternal risk factors for stillbirth such as advanced maternal age or obesity) [20]. Studies consistently report that the risk of stillbirth increases late in pregnancy, especially after 38 weeks of gestation. Elective induction at 39 weeks with prior history of stillbirth is recommended.

Management of pregnancy with previous stillbirth

Preconceptional/initial visit
Detailed history
Evaluation of prior stillbirth
Evaluate recurrence risk
Genetic counseling and screening

First trimester
Assess age by crown-rump length
Screen for diabetes
Folic acid supplementation

Second trimester
Screen for malformations (18-week ultrasonography)
Quadruple screening
Doppler assessment

Third trimester
Serial ultrasound (growth and biophysical profile) starting at 28 weeks of gestation
Antepartum fetal screening starting at 32–34 weeks

Delivery
Schedule elective delivery at 39 weeks
Individualize assessment for cases with multiple risk factors

Figure 6.1 Management of pregnancy with previous stillbirth.

POSTPARTUM CARE AFTER IUFD

Approaching a family for the autopsy of a stillbirth

Immediately following the stillbirth, families are often in a very intense grieving period and reference of autopsy at that time is often very painful to the family.

There is a high chance of refusal to provide consent for the procedure, and it is the right of the family to accept or reject the autopsy.

It is important to establish a rapport with the parents and take written consent for conducting an autopsy [4].

The following should be explained to the parents: the value of an autopsy, issues related to retained fetal tissues, the possibility that a cause may not be found, the appearance of the baby following autopsy, the likely time frame for results to become available, and arrangements for communicating results.

Karyotyping and cytogenic analysis

Experienced practitioners should inspect the baby when examining the infants. Rapid karyotyping utilizing quantitative fluorescent polymerase chain reaction (QF-PCR) or fluorescence *in situ* hybridization (FISH) can be used in difficult diagnoses.

Written consent is necessary prior to karyotyping with the use of samples from multiple tissues to increase the chance of culture. Multiple cytogenetic techniques can facilitate the chances of valuable results [4].

Support services and clinical counseling

The patient should be provided emotional support and adequate communication of test results [4].

The patient should be referred to a bereavement counselor, religious leader, support group, or mental health professional for management of grief and depression.

Suppression of lactation

The suppression of lactation is of psychological importance for some women following IUFD.

Pharmacologic measures are used to suppress lactation, preferably dopamine agonists, such as bromocriptine, cabergoline, and so on. [4].

Information about fertility and contraception

All women should be educated about the importance of contraception following IUFD to avoid psychological trauma.

Education and follow-up

Patients should be advised about the causes of late IUFD, risk of recurrence, and any measures to prevent further loss.

Counseling regarding smoking cessation, weight reduction, delayed conception until resolution of psychological trauma, and optimization of any other medical comorbidities [4].

CONCLUSION

- There are various causes of stillbirth, with unexplained stillbirth as the most common cause.
- Clinical assessment and laboratory tests should be offered to assess maternal well-being and the cause of stillbirth.
- For those women who chose expectant management, tests should be repeated twice a week (platelets and coagulation studies).
- If a woman is rhesus D negative, she should be offered anti-D as soon as possible after presentation.
- Continuation of expectant management versus delivery should be decided based on the medical condition of the patient.
- Those on prolonged expectant management should be advised that the value of fetal autopsy may be reduced.
- Vaginal birth is the target in most of the cases.
- Previous unexplained IUFD is an indication to recommend delivery at the specialist maternity unit, and most experts generally recommend elective induction at 39 weeks.

REFERENCES

1. World Health Organization. World Health Organization; Geneva, Switzerland: 2006. Neonatal and perinatal mortality country, regional and global estimates Barfield W. Clinical reports—Standard terminology for fetal, infant, and perinatal deaths. *Pediatrics*. 2011;128.
2. American College of Obstetricians and Gynecologists Management of Stillbirth. ACOG Practice Bulletin No. 102. *Obstet Gynecol*. 2009;113:748–61.
3. Royal College of Obstetricians and Gynaecologists. *Greentop Guideline 55— Late Intrauterine Fetal Death and Stillbirth*. London, UK: Royal College of Obstetricians and Gynaecologists; 2010.
4. Operational Guidelines for Establishing Sentinel Stillbirth Surveillance System, 2016 MOHFW, GOI.

5. Hoyert DL, Gregory ECW. *Cause of Fetal Death: Data from the Fetal Death Report, 2014. National Vital Statistics Reports*; Vol. 65, No. 7. Hyattsville, MD: National Center for Health Statistics; 2016.

6. Barfield WD, Committee on Fetus and Newborn. Standard terminology for fetal, infant, and perinatal deaths. *Pediatrics.* 2016;137.

7. Saleem S, Tikmani SS, McClure EM et al. Trends and determinants of stillbirth in developing countries: Results from the Global Network's Population-Based Birth Registry. *Reprod Health.* 2018;15(Suppl 1):100.

8. Aminu M, Bar-Zeev S, van den Broek N. Cause of and factors associated with stillbirth: A systematic review of classification systems. *Acta Obstet Gynecol Scand.* 2017;96:519.

9. Little SE, Zera CA, Clapp MA et al. A multistate analysis of early-term delivery trends and the association with term stillbirth. *Obstet Gynecol.* 2015;126:1138.

10. Dugoff L, Hobbins JC, Malone FD et al. First-trimester maternal serum PAPP-A and free-β subunit human chorionic gonadotropin concentrations and nuchal translucency are associated with obstetric complications: A population-based screening study (the FASTER Trial). *Am J Obstet Gynecol.* 2004;191:1446.

11. Fretts RC, Boyd ME, Usher RH, Usher HA. The changing pattern of fetal death, 1961–1988. *Obstet Gynecol.* 1992;79:35.

12. Pineles BL, Hsu S, Park E, Samet JM. Systematic review and meta-analyses of perinatal death and maternal exposure to tobacco smoke during pregnancy. *Am J Epidemiol.* 2016;184:87.

13. Goldenberg RL, McClure EM, Saleem S, Reddy UM. Infection-related stillbirths. *Lancet.* 2010;375:1482.

14. Gibbs RS. The origins of stillbirth: Infectious diseases. *Semin Perinatol.* 2002;26:75.

15. Groen H, Bouman K, Pierini A et al. Stillbirth and neonatal mortality in pregnancies complicated by major congenital anomalies: Findings from a large European cohort. *Prenat Diagn.* 2017;37:1100.

16. Clapp JF 3rd, Stepanchak W, Hashimoto K et al. The natural history of antenatal nuchal cords. *Am J Obstet Gynecol.* 2003;189:488.

17. Parasnis H, Raje B, Hinduja IN. Relevance of plasma fibrinogen estimation in obstetric complications. *J Postgrad Med.* 1992;38:183–5.

18. Wagaarachchi PT, Ashok PW, Narvekar NN, Smith NC, Templeton A. Medical management of late intrauterine death using a combination of mifepristone and misoprostol. *BJOG.* 2002;109:443–7.

19. Lawn JE, Blencowe H, Pattinson R et al. Stillbirths: Where? When? Why? How to make the data count? *Lancet.* 2011;377:1448.

20. Spong CY, Mercer BM, D'alton M et al. Timing of indicated late-preterm and early-term birth. *Obstet Gynecol.* 2011;118:323.

21. ACOG Practice Bulletin No. 102: Management of stillbirth. *Obstet Gynecol.* 2009;113:748. Reaffirmed 2019.

7

Investigation and management of recurrent cholestasis of pregnancy

SUJATA SIWATCH

INTRODUCTION

Intrahepatic cholestasis of pregnancy (ICP) has long been implicated as a rare cause of antepartum stillbirths, now being categorized under the Antepartum hypoxia category (A3) for the fetus and Maternal medical condition (M4) in the World Health Organization (WHO) application of the *International Classification of Diseases, 10th Revision,* to deaths during the perinatal period (*ICD–Perinatal Mortality, ICD-PM*) classification of stillbirths [1]. Intrahepatic cholestasis of pregnancy is a pregnancy-related liver disorder [2]. It usually presents in the second and third trimesters, though cases in the first trimester have also reported [3]. It is characterized by pruritis without a rash, especially on the palms and soles, that manifests itself more at night. A rise in bile acids is noted. This entity is characterized by a resolution of the symptoms and biochemical indicators after pregnancy. Cholestasis of pregnancy is associated with adverse fetal outcome, and so it is significant in women with previously unfavorable obstetric history. A history of recurrent cholestasis with jaundice and neonatal death should also be evaluated for genetic diseases, such as progressive familial intrahepatic cholestasis (PFIC) [4]. These women are also predisposed to develop various hepatobiliary, cardiovascular, and immune-mediated diseases in later life. The defining criteria and recommendations for management and delivery timing vary in the literature.

INCIDENCE/RECURRENCE

The incidence varies with ethnicity and region, suggesting a genetic, hormonal, and environmental influence in causation. The incidence in the United States is reported as 1%; in Chile, the reported incidence is 2.4%; and in Aracanos Indians, it is 5% [5]. The incidence in Indian Asians living in the United Kingdom is reported as 1.2%–1.5% [6]. It is known to recur in subsequent pregnancies (45%–90%) [6]. Cholelithiasis and women seropositive for hepatitis C virus (HCV) are considered risk factors by the American College of Obstetricians and Gynecologists (ACOG) and the Royal College of Obstetricians and Gynaecologists (RCOG) [2].

The risk of stillbirth due to cholestasis is true, but small. While it was reported as 107/1000 from 1965 to 1974 in an Australian center, its incidence reduced to 5.7/1000 in studies between 2001 and 2011, though the case selection and reporting bias still exist [7].

PREDISPOSITION

ICP is seen more commonly in Chile, Southeast Asia, South America, and Scandinavian countries. Though the exact etiopathogenesis is uncertain, it also plays an important role [8]. Women with sensitivity to estrogen-containing contraceptives are predisposed to develop ICP in pregnancy. Pregnancy with multiple gestations is associated with a higher rate of cholestasis. Increases in its severity are reported in the winter months.

Genetic factors have been implicated in the development of ICP. Various genes have been implicated in its causation, the most literature being on ABCC and MDR3 genes that are related to the secretion and transport of bile salts and lipids. The clinical presentation of genetic predisposition ranges from PFIC to benign recurrent intrahepatic cholestasis (BRIC) to ICP [4,9].

PATHOPHYSIOLOGY

ICP is characterized by pruritis without any other skin lesions. There is a rise in the serum levels of bile salts, especially taurocholate and taurodeoxycholic acids [8], that deposit under the surface of the skin leading to itching. The defect is thought to cause loss of function of secretion and transport of bile salts from the liver, leading to a rise in serum bile salts. Pregnancy is a state with highly elevated levels of estrogen, progesterone, and corticosteroids, which further precipitate the cholestasis by inhibiting the bile salt export pump of the hepatocytes and impairing sulfation [10].

It is postulated that the taurocholate crosses the placenta to the fetus and may cause fetal arrythmias and increase the PR interval. A few animal studies have also suggested the same. Some authors also suggest that exposure to increased bile salts leads to sudden constriction of the human chorionic vein. This may lead to fetal distress and sudden fetal demise.

DIFFERENTIALS

The diagnostic criteria of ICP are not clearly defined; ICP is basically a diagnosis of exclusion. Pruritis is present in 23% of pregnancies [11], though the prevalence of cholestasis of pregnancy is much lower. Other dermatologic conditions like scabies, pemphigoid gestationis, prurigo of pregnancy, pruritic folliculitis of pregnancy, Pityrosporum folliculitis, pustular folliculitis, benign pruritis gravidarum, skin allergies, and other chronic diseases need to be ruled out, especially with skin lesions [12]. Scratch marks may be found on the skin. Other than that, liver disorders with raised liver enzymes need to be considered, including viral hepatitis, gallstone disease, acute fatty liver of pregnancy, and even preeclampsia.

EFFECT ON MORBIDITY/ MORTALITY—MATERNAL/ NEONATAL

Although ICP causes few maternal concerns, it influences fetal and neonatal morbidity and mortality and thus is significant, especially in women with previous pregnancy losses.

For the mother, ICP may cause maternal distress attributable to intense itching that may be mild or even severe enough to cause suicidal ideation due to disturbed night sleep and poor quality of life. Skin scarring and secondary infections may also result. Vitamin K deficiency may be caused due to fat malabsorption and steatorrhea and thus is thought to predispose to postpartum hemorrhage, though few studies report it [13].

The fetal effects are more unsettling. ICP is associated with a higher rate of stillbirth, prematurity, meconium-stained liquor, fetal distress, and sudden fetal demise. In an observational study from a tertiary care hospital in North India, a total of 15 stillbirths (0.4% of 3678 total from 2008 to 2017) have been attributed to cholestasis [14]. Moreover, surveillance tools cannot help predict the timings of these adverse outcomes. The complications increase with advancing gestation.

In a recent systematic literature review and meta-analysis published by Ovadia et al., the associations of adverse perinatal outcomes of ICP with biochemical markers were studied [15]. ICP was associated with a stillbirth rate of 0.91% (45 of 4936 cases) as compared to 0.32% (519 of 163,947 controls). The odds ratio of stillbirth in singleton pregnancies was 1.46, though with significant study heterogeneity.

The stillbirth rate correlated with a serum maximum total bile acid concentration (AUROC 0.83 [95% CI 0.74–0.92]) [15]. However, no significant association was found with levels of alanine aminotransferase (AUROC 0.46 [95% CI 0.35–0.57]), aspartate aminotransferase (AUROC 0.58 [0.33–0.83]), or bilirubin (AUROC 0.79 [0.62–0.92]). The serum bile acid levels were studied in three groups—less than 40, 40–99 mcgmol/L, and more than 100 mcgmol/L. The stillbirth risk was significantly increased in the latter group with a 30.5 hazard ratio as compared to the women with less than 40 mcgmol/L. The stillbirth rates of women with levels less than 40 mcgmol/L were comparable to the general population. Fortunately, the majority of women with ICP have bile acids of less than 40 μmol/L.

Premature birth, both spontaneous and iatrogenic, was higher in the ICP cases than in controls. Though iatrogenic prematurity contributed significantly to the overall premature deliveries at all serum levels of total bile acid, even spontaneous-onset preterm deliveries were higher, especially in women with serum bile acid levels more than 100 μmol/L. The odds ratio was 3.47 (95% CI 3.06–3.95) for the spontaneous group and 3.65 (95% CI 1.94–6.85) for the iatrogenic group [15]. Most women with multiple gestation also delivered preterm.

Women with ICP are more likely to have meconium-stained liquor (odds ratio 2.6 [1.6–4.1]) [15]. The babies of these women were more likely to be admitted in the neonatal care unit (odds ratio 2.12 [1.48–3.03]) but have similar birth weight. Lee et al. suggested that there is a 19.7% increase in the risk of meconium passage with each 10 μmol/L rising level of total bile acid concentration ($p = .001$) [13]. The rate of cesarean sections is also higher (ranging 0%–36%), which can be contributed by early induction, patient anxiety, or cholestasis [16].

Other than higher levels of bile acids, according to Shan et al. and Mei et al., adverse perinatal outcomes increase with earlier onset of ICP [17,18].

PROGRESSIVE FAMILIAL INTRAHEPATIC CHOLESTASIS

PFIC (further divided into types 1–5), BRIC, and ICP are a spectrum of genetic liver diseases that may present with cholestasis in pregnancy [4,9]. ICP is the most benign form, with self-limiting disease presenting in pregnancy, with low fetal morbidity and mortality, especially with good obstetrical surveillance and management. On the other side of the spectrum, PFIC 1 and 2 are more sinister expressions that present as neonatal jaundice that progresses to liver cirrhosis and failure. BRIC is a milder intermittent presentation that is mostly nonprogressive (Table 7.1) [4]. When suspected, prenatal genetic analysis with amniocentesis can be done after appropriate counseling [19]. These rare hereditary cholestases have an autosomal recessive inheritance pattern.

INVESTIGATIONS

Bile salts, especially taurocholate and taurodeoxycholate, are implicated in the pathogenesis of ICP. According to the American College of Gastroenterologists, the European Association for the Study of the Liver, and the Society of Maternal-Fetal Medicine, a fasting bile acid level of more than 10 μ/dL is considered as a cutoff to make a diagnosis of cholestasis of pregnancy along with persistent itching that improves after the pregnancy [20–23]. Bile acid levels rise after intake of food, so diagnosing cholestasis of pregnancy by fasting levels may lead to underdiagnosis of some patients. Random levels are generally used in clinical practice [16]. The diagnosis of ICP is not excluded by normal levels of bile salts. The rise of bilirubin levels may be seen, but levels are usually low (less than 5 mg/dL) and develop weeks after the pruritis. Transaminitis is also seen. Pregnancy-specific cutoffs for liver function test levels should be considered, which are usually 20% lower for transaminases, bilirubin, and γ-glutamyl transferase [16].

The diagnosis of ICP requires exclusion of other causes of cholestasis including drug intake, gallstone disease, autoimmune disorders, and viral hepatitis [8]. An ultrasound of the liver and gallbladder and viral markers are thus required. Preeclampsia and acute fatty liver of pregnancy may present with raised transaminases and thus the diagnosis should also be considered and excluded. Dermatologic disorders like scabies may also mimic ICP by causing pruritus. A dermatologic opinion should thus be taken to rule them out.

ICP has been associated with a higher prevalence of gestational diabetes and even preeclampsia [24].

Table 7.1 Differences between PFIC (progressive familial intrahepatic cholestasis), BRIC (benign recurrent intrahepatic cholestasis), and ICP (intrahepatic cholestasis of pregnancy)

	PFIC	BRIC	ICP
Types	PFIC 1–5	BRIC 1, 2	ICP 1–3
Gene mutation	ATP8B1 deficiency, ABCBC11, ABCB4, MDR3, TJP2	ATP8B1, ABCB11	ABCB4, ABCB11, ATP8B1
Presentation	Variable, infancy to adulthood	Usually after first decade	In second or third trimester of pregnancy
Course of disease	Permanent, generally progressive	Episodic attacks of variable duration (weeks to months)	Transient cholestasis in pregnancy with postpartum resolution
Management	UDCA, rifampicin, cholestyramine, surgery—biliary diversion, liver transplantation	Rifampicin, cholestyramine, nasobiliary drainage, plasmapheresis	UDCA may help pruritis, prenatal/intrapartum surveillance, termination of pregnancy after 37 weeks
Adverse outcomes	Cirrhosis, cancers—hepatocellular carcinoma or cholangiocarcinoma		Stillbirths, fetal distress, meconium-stained liquor

Thus, women with ICP must also be evaluated for gestational diabetes. A coagulation screen should also be done as steatorrhea may cause a deficiency of vitamin K absorption that is required for the formation of coagulation factors.

MANAGEMENT

A woman with a history of cholestasis of pregnancy should be counseled regarding the recurrence of cholestasis in pregnancy and its potential effects on the mother and the fetus so that she can be vigilant of the symptoms. After the diagnosis of ICP, the management includes therapy to alleviate the maternal symptoms of itching and prevention of adverse fetal/neonatal outcome (Figure 7.1). Women with a family history or history of a neonatal death with jaundice, pruritis, hepatosplenomegaly, especially with a history of consanguinity and cholestasis of pregnancy, may be considered for prenatal testing. DNA analysis of both parents may show heterozygous mutations. The role of noninvasive prenatal testing is still limited. Amniocentesis and DNA analysis may help in the prenatal diagnosis of PFIC and help parents with affected fetuses to make a decision for termination of pregnancy. Monitoring of the pregnancy includes serial one to two times per week monitoring of the liver function tests

[16]. Spontaneous normalization of the levels on subsequent monitoring reduces the chances of diagnosis of cholestasis of pregnancy. Blood pressure and urine albumin should be done to rule out preeclampsia. Rapidly increasing LFTs may also point to an alternative diagnosis [16]. LFTs should be repeated in the postpartum period after 10 days postpartum as LFTs may increase initially in the early puerperium [25]. A normalization of the LFTs is seen in ICP, while raised levels point to alternative diagnoses, like autoimmune disease that should be further evaluated. The South Australian Maternal and Neonatal Community of Practice (SAMNCP) recommends that women with bile acids >40 mcmol/L or ALT >200 IU/L be admitted and biweekly bile acid tests and LFTs be done. Outpatient management is acceptable if medications lower the ALT and bile acids to below threshold [26].

RCOG recommends booking these patients for "consultant-led care" and hospital deliveries [16]. The role of careful obstetrical fetal surveillance needs special emphasis. However, no fetal monitoring has been shown to predict fetal demise. The suggested fetal monitoring includes biweekly biophysical profile and nonstress test. The role of maternal daily fetal movement count cannot be overemphasized. There is no evidence of fetal growth restriction or placental insufficiency with

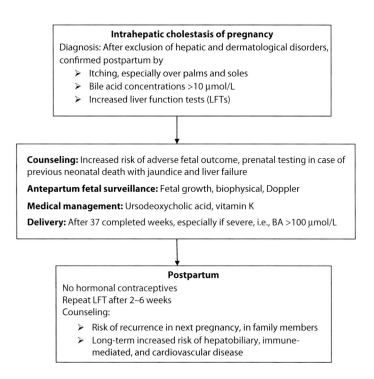

Intrahepatic cholestasis of pregnancy
Diagnosis: After exclusion of hepatic and dermatological disorders, confirmed postpartum by
- Itching, especially over palms and soles
- Bile acid concentrations >10 μmol/L
- Increased liver function tests (LFTs)

Counseling: Increased risk of adverse fetal outcome, prenatal testing in case of previous neonatal death with jaundice and liver failure

Antepartum fetal surveillance: Fetal growth, biophysical, Doppler

Medical management: Ursodeoxycholic acid, vitamin K

Delivery: After 37 completed weeks, especially if severe, i.e., BA >100 μmol/L

Postpartum
No hormonal contraceptives
Repeat LFT after 2–6 weeks
Counseling:
- Risk of recurrence in next pregnancy, in family members
- Long-term increased risk of hepatobiliary, immune-mediated, and cardiovascular disease

Figure 7.1 Diagnosis and management of ICP in pregnancy.

Doppler, similar to other pregnancies. Various scientific bodies recommend that the decision for termination of pregnancy after 37 completed weeks should be made with the patient after prior counseling [21–23,26,27].

Termination of pregnancy should be planned after due discussion with the patient [16]. Women with cholestasis should be advised of the small increase in the risk of stillbirth if pregnancy continues, that the risk increases with rising bile acid levels, and that it may be sudden and cannot be predicted. Conversely, the higher perinatal morbidity due to early delivery and maternal morbidity due to induction of labor should be discussed. The risk of admission of the baby to the special care unit following elective cesarean sections is reported as –11%, 6%, and 1.5% at 37, 38, and 39 weeks of gestation, though the same may vary in different centers [28]. In twin gestation, stillbirth in ICP and twin pregnancy occurs at 33–35 weeks [29], the rate increasing with levels of bile acids, and is speculated to be associated with gestational diabetes [30]. This pregnancy may thus be terminated at around 36 weeks' gestation.

Use of emollients like coconut oil, calamine lotion, and aqueous cream with menthol are among many bland topical applications that may be helpful [16].

Various medications have been used in cholestasis of pregnancy. The drugs that have been used for pruritis include antihistaminics like chlorphenamine that help alleviate the itching by causing sedation at night. Cholestyramine, a bile acid chelating agent, helps improve pruritis but increases vitamin K deficiency. Activated charcoal and guar gum are not helpful. In addition, S-adenosyl methionine (SAMe) has not been found to be useful in relieving itching or improving perinatal outcome. The reports of usefulness of dexamethasone are controversial and not recommended. Other drugs like rifampicin and metformin have been reportedly used as adjunctive medications for ICP that are refractory to ursodiol alone [31].

Ursodeoxycholic acid (UDCA) has been used widely for ICP, though its role is not clear. A Cochrane review, though restricted by the absence of large good quality studies, indicated that UDCA may help in reducing maternal pruritis, but it does not have a role in reducing adverse perinatal outcomes [32,33]. In the PITCHES trial, which was a double-blind, multicentric randomized controlled trial in England and Wales, the effect of UDCA was studied versus placebo, to compare a composite of perinatal death, preterm delivery, and neonatal unit admission [34]. They concluded that UDCA does not improve an adverse perinatal outcome rate in women with ICP.

Vitamin K may be administered to prevent coagulation factor deficiency due to steatorrhea leading to malabsorption of fat-soluble vitamin K. It is recommended in oral water-soluble form (menadiol sodium phosphate) in 5–10 mg doses daily, if prothrombin time is prolonged, to reduce the risk of postpartum hemorrhage and bleeding in the neonate [15]. If normal, the side effects should be considered before it is recommended. Due to the risk of kernicterus, neonatal hemolytic anemia, and hyperbilirubinemia, the British National Formulary has advised to refrain from vitamin K therapy in late pregnancy and labor. Newborn babies may be given vitamin K as usual [16].

POSTPARTUM

LFTs should be repeated only after 10 days, as there may be a transient increase in the enzyme levels in the postpartum period [25]. The woman should be counseled regarding the repetition in later pregnancies and higher chances of cholestasis in members of the family. Estrogen-containing oral contraceptives are contraindicated. Progesterone-containing contraceptives, however, can be taken.

CONCLUSION

- Pruritis, raised bile acids, and LFTs are characteristic features of ICP.
- The prevalence of cholestasis of pregnancy varies and is linked to genetic predisposition, ethnicity, multiple gestation, and winter months. Recurrence rates are between 45% and 90%.
- It is associated with poor perinatal outcomes including stillbirths, which are sudden and unpredictable.
- Bile acid value greater than 100 μmol/L is associated with poor perinatal outcomes.
- Fetal surveillance and early term delivery are advocated.
- Genetic causes are rare but should be considered with previously unfavorable obstetric history.

REFERENCES

1. Allanson ER, Tuncalp Ö, Gardosi J et al. Giving a voice to millions: Developing the WHO application of *ICD-10* to deaths during the perinatal period: *ICD-PM. BJOG.* 2016;123(12):1896–9.
2. Bicocca MJ, Sperling JD, Chauhan SP. Intrahepatic cholestasis of pregnancy: Review of six national and regional guidelines. *Eur J Obstet Gynecol Reprod Biol.* 2018;231:180–7.
3. Hubschmann AG, Orzechowski KM, Berghella V. Severe first trimester recurrent intrahepatic cholestasis of pregnancy: A case report and literature review. *AJP Rep.* 2016;6(1):e38–41.
4. Srivastava A. Progressive familial intrahepatic cholestasis. *J Clin Exp Hepatol.* 2014;4(1):25–36.
5. Reyes H, Gonzalez MC, Ribalta J et al. Prevalence of intrahepatic cholestasis of pregnancy in Chile. *Ann Intern Med.* 1978;88(4):487–93.
6. Abedin P, Weaver JB, Egginton E. Intrahepatic cholestasis of pregnancy: Prevalence and ethnic distribution. *Ethnicity Health.* 1999;4(1–2):35–7.
7. Reid R, Ivey KJ, Rencoret RH, Storey B. Fetal complications of obstetric cholestasis. *Br Med J.* 1976;1(6014):870–2.
8. Ozkan S, Ceylan Y, Ozkan OV, Yildirim S. Review of a challenging clinical issue: Intrahepatic cholestasis of pregnancy. *World J Gastroenterol.* 2015;21(23):7134–41.
9. Sticova E, Jirsa M, Pawlowska J. New insights in genetic cholestasis: From molecular mechanisms to clinical implications. *Can J Gastroenterol Hepatol.* 2018;2018:2313675.
10. Lammert F, Marschall HU, Glantz A, Matern S. Intrahepatic cholestasis of pregnancy: Molecular pathogenesis, diagnosis and management. *J Hepatol.* 2000;33(6):1012–21.
11. Kenyon AP, Tribe RM, Nelson-Piercy C et al. Pruritus in pregnancy: A study of anatomical distribution and prevalence in relation to the development of obstetric cholestasis. *Obstet Med.* 2010;3(1):25–9.
12. Chao TT, Sheffield JS. Primary dermatologic findings with early-onset intrahepatic cholestasis of pregnancy. *Obstet Gynecol.* 2011;117(2 Pt 2):456–8.

13. Lee RH, Kwok KM, Ingles S et al. Pregnancy outcomes during an era of aggressive management for intrahepatic cholestasis of pregnancy. *Am J Perinatol.* 2008;25(6):341–5.

14. Sharma B, Prasad G, Aggarwal N, Siwatch S, Suri V, Kakkar N. Aetiology and trends of rates of stillbirth in a tertiary care hospital in the north of India over 10 years: A retrospective study. *BJOG.* 2019;126(Suppl. 4):14–20.

15. Ovadia C, Seed PT, Sklavounos A et al. Association of adverse perinatal outcomes of intrahepatic cholestasis of pregnancy with biochemical markers: Results of aggregate and individual patient data meta-analyses. *Lancet.* 2019;393(10174):899–909.

16. Royal College of Obstetricians and Gynaecologists. *Obstetric Cholestasis. RCOG Green-top Guideline No. 43.* London, UK: RCOG; 2011.

17. Mei Y, Lin Y, Luo D, Gao L, He L. Perinatal outcomes in intrahepatic cholestasis of pregnancy with monochorionic diamniotic twin pregnancy. *BMC Pregnancy Childbirth.* 2018;18(1):291.

18. Shan D, Hu Y, Qiu P et al. Intrahepatic cholestasis of pregnancy in women with twin pregnancy. *Twin Res Human Genet.* 2016;19(6):697–707.

19. Chen ST, Chen HL, Su YN et al. Prenatal diagnosis of progressive familial intrahepatic cholestasis type 2. *J Gastroenterol Hepatol.* 2008; 23(9):1390–3.

20. Egan N, Bartels A, Khashan AS et al. Reference standard for serum bile acids in pregnancy. *BJOG.* 2012;119(4):493–8.

21. EASL Clinical Practice Guidelines: Management of cholestatic liver diseases. *J Hepatol.* 2009;51(2):237–67.

22. Publications Committee Society of Maternal-Fetal Medicine. Understanding Intrahepatic Cholestasis of Pregnancy. 2011. https://www.smfm.org/publications/96-understanding-intrahepatic-cholestasis-of-pregnancy. Accessed September 10, 2017.

23. Tran TT, Ahn J, Reau NS. ACG clinical guideline: Liver disease and pregnancy. *Am J Gastroenterol.* 2016;111(2):176–94; quiz 96.

24. Wikstrom Shemer E, Marschall HU, Ludvigsson JF, Stephansson O. Intrahepatic cholestasis of pregnancy and associated adverse pregnancy and fetal outcomes: A 12-year population-based cohort study. *BJOG.* 2013;120(6):717–23.

25. David AL, Kotecha M, Girling JC. Factors influencing postnatal liver function tests. *BJOG.* 2000;107(11):1421–6.

26. South Australian Maternal and Neonatal Community of Practice. *Obstetric Cholestasis;* 2016.

27. Rioseco AJ, Ivankovic MB, Manzur A et al. Intrahepatic cholestasis of pregnancy: A retrospective case-control study of perinatal outcome. *Am J Obstet Gynecol.* 1994; 170(3):890–5.

28. Morrison JJ, Rennie JM, Milton PJ. Neonatal respiratory morbidity and mode of delivery at term: Influence of timing of elective caesarean section. *Br J Obstet Gynaecol.* 1995;102(2):101–6.

29. Liu X, Landon MB, Chen Y, Cheng W. Perinatal outcomes with intrahepatic cholestasis of pregnancy in twin pregnancies. *J Matern Fetal Neonatal Med.* 2016;29(13):2176–81.

30. Shaw D, Frohlich J, Wittmann BA, Willms M. A prospective study of 18 patients with cholestasis of pregnancy. *Am J Obstet Gynecol.* 1982;142(6 Pt 1):621–5.

31. Elfituri A, Ali A, Shehata H. Managing recurring obstetric cholestasis with metformin. *Obstet Gynecol.* 2016;128(6):1320–3.

32. Gurung V, Middleton P, Milan SJ, Hague W, Thornton JG. Interventions for treating cholestasis in pregnancy. *Cochrane Database Syst Rev.* 2013;(6):CD000493. doi: 10.1002/14651858.CD000493.

33. Mishra N, Rohilla M. Intrahepatic cholestasis of pregnancy: Advances in diagnosis and management. *J Gynecol* 2017; 2(S3): S3-0005.

34. Chappell LC, Bell JL, Smith A et al. Ursodeoxycholic acid versus placebo in women with intrahepatic cholestasis of pregnancy (PITCHES): A randomised controlled trial. *Lancet.* 2019;394(10201):849–60.

8

Management of women with prior hypertension and abruptio placentae in pregnancy

SHALINI GAINDER AND DEEPMALA MODI

INTRODUCTION

Certain diseases in pregnancy have an impact on the current pregnancy to make it high risk, may also predict the risk of a woman developing certain disorders in the future, and may also have an impact in future pregnancies. There is enough evidence to suggest that there is recurrence of hypertension in pregnancy. Hypertension-related disorders in pregnancy continue to be the leading causes of maternal and perinatal morbidity and mortality and affect 10% of pregnancies worldwide. Approximately 50,000–60,000 deaths related to preeclampsia are reported worldwide [1,2]. Hypertension leads to various complications and is a major contributor of prematurity. Identifying the patient and diagnosing preeclampsia are a major clinical challenge. Imparting the education to patients and implementing various counseling strategies are needed for early detection of hypertensive disorders in subsequent pregnancies for women who are affected in previous pregnancy.

Preeclampsia syndrome includes the development of hypertension in the latter half of pregnancy associated with new-onset proteinuria, although it is not an essential criterion for diagnosis [3]. Other clinical signs suggestive of disease may also be present.

"Diagnostic criteria include the development of hypertension, defined as a persistent systolic blood pressure (BP) of 140 mm Hg or higher, or a diastolic BP of 90 mm Hg or higher after 20 weeks of gestation in a women with previously normal blood pressure" [4].

Hypertension in pregnancy is further divided into four categories:

1. Gestational hypertension
2. Preeclampsia–eclampsia

3. Chronic hypertension (primary or secondary)
4. Chronic hypertension with superimposed pre-eclampsia [5]

The primary goal in women with previous pre-eclampsia is to decrease the risk factors causing recurrence, optimize maternal health prior to conception, confirm early diagnosis of preeclampsia and its complications in subsequent pregnancies, and achieve optimal perinatal outcome. To achieve this goal, preconceptional counseling, early booking in prenatal period, adequate prenatal visits, maternal and fetal surveillance, timely referral, and institutional delivery are required.

RISK OF RECURRENCE OF HYPERTENSION IN PREGNANCY

The overall risk of recurrence in future pregnancies in women with hypertensive disorders of pregnancy is approximately one in five women (Table 8.1).

Recurrence in gestational hypertension: In women with gestational hypertension in previous pregnancy, the prevalence of gestational hypertension is 11%–15% (up to one in seven women) and preeclampsia is 7% (1 in 14 women) in a future pregnancy. The risk of development of chronic hypertension is 3% (up to 1 in 34 women) in subsequent pregnancy.

Recurrence in preeclampsia: In women with previous preeclampsia, the future risk of gestational hypertension is 6%–12% (up to one in eight women) and preeclampsia is 16% (one in six women).

Previous early-onset preeclampsia: The risk of preeclampsia further increases to 23% (one in four women) for women who gave birth at 34–37 weeks in previous pregnancy and to 33% (one in three women) for women who gave birth at 28–34 weeks. The risk of development of chronic hypertension is 2% (up to 1 in 50 women) in subsequent pregnancies [6–8].

Women with previous early onset preeclampsia are considered as a separate group with increased chances of recurrence. Likely underlying causes of hypertension including antiphospholipid syndrome or thrombophilias should be evaluated and the possibility of undiagnosed chronic hypertension or renal disorder have to be considered.

PRECONCEPTIONAL COUNSELING

Preconceptional counseling prior to the next pregnancy is recommended in women with preeclampsia in previous pregnancy and should be done ideally at a visit before the next pregnancy is planned. But if the woman seems unlikely to comply with attending a preconception visit, then the assessment findings done at 6–8 weeks postpartum would be considered as baseline.

At this visit, a detailed history of previous pregnancy should be taken. All the prenatal, intrapartum, and postpartum events must be meticulously recorded. The medical records available must be screened for information like gestation at which there was onset of preeclampsia, development of maternal complications like preeclampsia, or worsening of the disease. Perinatal outcome must also be recorded to check for previous fetal growth restriction and perinatal morbidity and mortality [9,10]. The risk of recurrence and its impact on subsequent pregnancy must be discussed with the couple. The effect of pregnancy on hypertensive disorders and the effect of hypertension/preeclampsia on perinatal outcome must be discussed. The woman should also be told that the risk of recurrence increases further if the interpregnancy interval is more than 10 years.

Evaluation of associated risk factors like history of infertility and comorbidities like obesity, kidney disease, chronic hypertension, diabetes mellitus, connective tissue disorders, and thrombophilia and antiphospholipid syndrome should

Table 8.1 Risk of recurrence of hypertension in subsequent pregnancy

Prevalence in future pregnancy	Any hypertension (%)	Gestational hypertension (%)	Preeclampsia (%)
Any hypertension	21	22	20
Preeclampsia	14	7	16
Gestational hypertension	9	11–15	6–12
Chronic hypertension	Not applicable	3	2

also be done [11]. Routine screening for thrombophilia is not recommended in women with prior preeclampsia, but some clinics still include this in the workup of women with past hypertension in pregnancy. The underlying disease status should be optimized prior to conception, and strict control of the disease and glycemic control must be ensured. Attempts should be made to reduce the modifiable risk factors like weight loss in women with increased body mass index (BMI), increasing physical activity and adopting a healthy lifestyle. Overweight women should be counseled on the potential benefits of weight reduction and must be given nutritional counseling [12].

Various laboratory investigations, i.e., baseline complete blood count, metabolic profile, renal function test, and urinalysis may be done for evaluation of the disease and its complications. Medications being taken by the patient for any preexisting disorder must be reviewed and may be changed as per their teratogenic potential and U.S. Food and Drug Administration category status. Women should be advised to visit the health-care practitioner early when found to be pregnant.

Preconceptional administration of folic acid is recommended.

ANTEPARTUM MANAGEMENT

In a patient with a previous history of preeclampsia, early booking is advisable.

Early first-trimester ultrasound must be done for accurate assessment of gestational age. The frequency of further prenatal visits must be determined as per previous pregnancy outcomes. The woman with previous early-onset preeclampsia or the one resulting in preterm delivery must have earlier and more frequent health checkup visits. The woman should be informed about the signs and symptoms of preeclampsia and its prodromal features. Therefore, risk stratification can be done based on previous gestation.

Baseline laboratory investigations like complete blood count, renal function tests, metabolic profile, and urinalysis should be done at the first trimester. In women with previous early-onset preeclampsia, renal ultrasound can be considered, and thrombophilia screening is routinely done by some clinics.

It has been studied that systemic prostacyclin-thromboxane balance is altered in preeclampsia [13]. Low-dose aspirin (60–80 mg daily dose) is started in the late first trimester if preeclampsia in previous pregnancy led to the delivery of a preterm infant (less than 34 0/7 weeks) or if the woman had recurrent preeclampsia in more than one pregnancy [14,15]. The use of low-dose aspirin was studied in a meta-analysis of 59 studies comprising 37,000 women, and this indicated its potential benefit in high-risk women for reducing preeclampsia incidence and its adverse perinatal outcomes [16].

In the second trimester, reinforce information about signs and symptoms of preeclampsia, which may be supplemented by printed handouts. Instructions must be given to report if symptoms like severe headache, visual disturbances, nausea and vomiting, right upper quadrant or epigastrium discomfort and pain, or decreased fetal movements occur. Blood pressure should be checked at every prenatal visit, and the patient should also be advised to maintain home blood pressure records. The patient should be monitored for signs of preeclampsia at every visit.

Hospital admission is advocated for preeclampsia with severe features, severe fetal growth restriction, and recurrent preeclampsia for frequent maternal and fetal surveillance.

The frequency of both maternal and fetal surveillance must be increased in the last trimester as indicated. Daily assessment of maternal symptoms and fetal movement should be done by the patient. Since there is a known correlation between fetal growth restriction and preeclampsia, laboratory parameters, serial ultrasonography for fetal growth restriction and amniotic fluid assessment, umbilical artery Doppler, biophysical profile, and nonstress test must be done as indicated [17].

POSTPARTUM MANAGEMENT

There should be inpatient or equivalent outpatient monitoring of blood pressure for at least 72 hours postpartum. It should be checked again at 1 week after delivery or earlier if the woman has symptoms. Discharge advice should include information about signs and symptoms of preeclampsia and severe features. Nonsteroidal anti-inflammatory drugs for pain relief must be avoided if the hypertension persists beyond 1 day postpartum.

Antihypertensive therapy in the postpartum period is recommended if the systolic blood pressure is more than 150 mm Hg or the diastolic equal to or more than 100 mm Hg on two occasions at least 4 hours apart [18,19].

Blood pressure should be rechecked at 6–8 weeks postpartum. If the woman has no hypertension or proteinuria at this visit, she should be told that the absolute risk of development of chronic renal disease is less, and a further follow-up is not necessary although relative risk is slightly higher.

FUTURE CARDIOVASCULAR DISEASE IN WOMEN WITH PREVIOUS PREECLAMPSIA

After various research and studies, it has been concluded that women who develop preeclampsia in pregnancy have an increased predisposition (up to two times) to develop cardiovascular disorders in later life (Table 8.2). The risk further escalates to eight- to ninefold in women in whom preeclampsia led to premature delivery before 34 0/7 weeks of gestation [20–22] or women with recurrent preeclampsia [23]. These women have increased risk of developing chronic hypertension, stroke, congestive heart failure, and myocardial infarction.

The exact mechanism of this correlation with cardiovascular disease is not yet well understood, but it has been observed that the endothelial dysfunction which is also associated with atherosclerosis persists for many years after a pregnancy is affected by preeclampsia. It has been postulated that 50% of increased risk of development of future chronic hypertension or cardiovascular morbidities can be explained by the prepregnancy common risk factors [24]. It has also been stated that preeclampsia might trigger a biological response that leads to cardiovascular stress that would not have taken place otherwise, despite the presence of risk factors or genetic predisposition.

The American Heart Association advocates that the obstetric history should be an important component of history while evaluating cardiovascular risks in women [25]. It is presumed that preeclampsia and cardiovascular disease have common risk factors. Weight reduction, increased physical activity, smoking cessation, and early evaluation of cardiovascular risks are recommended in women who had preeclampsia.

In women with a history of preeclampsia leading to preterm delivery or delivery of a baby with fetal growth restriction, or a history of recurrent preeclampsia, it is recommended that blood pressure, fasting blood sugar levels, lipid profiles, and BMI should be assessed every year. These women should be further advised to maintain ideal body weight. A diet that is high in fiber, fruits, and vegetables and low in fat is recommended. It is advisable to do aerobic exercise at least five times per week. They should also be instructed to avoid alcohol, smoking, and tobacco.

WOMEN WITH PLACENTAL ABRUPTION IN PREVIOUS PREGNANCY

Placental abruption (PA) is a major cause of perinatal mortality occurring in some women without predictable causes. It has an impact on reproductive behavior. A woman following placental abruption in previous pregnancy should be considered high risk, not only because of recurrence of abruption but there is also an increased risk of small for gestational age infant, preterm birth, and pregnancy-induced hypertension (PIH) both in recurrent abruption cases and in subsequent non-PA deliveries [26,27].

PREDICTION OF ABRUPTION

Abruption without hypertension associated with the pregnancy is termed as *nontoxemic abruption*, and when pregnancy-associated or underlying chronic hypertension is present in a woman, then the placental abruption is termed as *toxemic abruption*.

The risk factors have been studied by various epidemiological studies [28–33]. Abruption in a

Table 8.2 Cardiovascular risk in women with hypertensive disorder in previous pregnancy

Risk	Gestational hypertension	Preeclampsia	Chronic hypertension
Cardiovascular event	1.5–3 times	1.5–3 times	1.7 times
Stroke	2 times	2–3 times	1.8 times
Hypertension	2–4 times	2–5 times	Not applicable

previous pregnancy is the most important factor in predicting its recurrence in the next pregnancy. Recurrence of abruption is 4% after abruption in one previous pregnancy [34], and it increases to 19%–25% for women who had two previous pregnancies that were complicated by abruption [35].

VARIOUS OTHER RISK FACTORS

The following are other risk factors for PA.

Maternal: Advanced age, multiparity, low BMI, maternal thrombophilia (especially heterozygous factor V Leiden and heterozygous prothrombin 20210A) [36,37], pregnancies following assisted reproductive technology (ART), first-trimester bleeding or threatened abortion [38], preeclampsia, chronic hypertension, polyhydramnios, intrauterine infection, premature rupture of membranes, abdominal trauma, smoking, and drug abuse (amphetamine and cocaine).

Fetal: Fetal growth restriction and nonvertex presentation are fetal risk factors for recurrence of PA. In women with PA, there was an increased risk of recurrence in women with a history of preterm birth associated with SGA baby in the immediate previous delivery with as high as three times increased risk of PA, while women who had hypertension in the previous pregnancy, but not in the current, had a 60% increased risk of PA [27].

Therefore, all pregnant women must be screened for these risk factors at each prenatal visit. Thereby, women should be designated as high-risk or low-risk pregnancies; however, 70% of placental abruptions occur in low-risk pregnancies.

In a study comprising 1,570,635 women, 3496 (0.22%) women developed PA. It was found that the risk of PA was significantly higher in women who had PA in previous pregnancy (5.8%) as compared to women without abruption in previous pregnancy (0.06%). The risk of recurrence was further increased if the previous abruption occurred at term as compared to previous preterm abruption.

Recurrence of abruptio placentae in normotensive versus hypertensive pregnancies: PA was more frequent in hypertensive women (0.44% versus 0.16%) as compared to normotensive women. The recurrence of abruption in hypertensive women was less than in normotensive women [39].

In the recent literature, it was suggested that since the incidence of recurrence of hypertension in pregnancy decreases in second pregnancy, the recurrence of toxemic abruptio is much less compared to normotensive pregnancies. This risk cannot be extrapolated to women with chronic hypertension where the recurrence is about 9% and increases to 20% when there is associated superimposed preeclampsia. The true recurrence of abruptio cannot be defined as most pregnancies are terminated electively at 37 weeks; therefore, whether these would have recurred is not known.

PREVENTION OF ABRUPTION

Women should be advised and encouraged to change the modifiable risk factors such as smoking and drug misuse.

A systemic review regarding folic acid intake during pregnancy has failed to find any benefit in reducing the risk of abruption [40]. Similarly, there is lack of evidence and data to support the use of antithrombotic therapy (low-dose aspirin or low molecular weight aspirin) in preventing abruption in women with thrombophilia [41].

In a pilot study in women with a previous PA, it was found that the women who received enoxaparin in subsequent pregnancy had lesser placenta-related vascular complications like preeclampsia, abruption, or low birth weight [42], although large multicentric trials are needed to validate the finding.

MANAGEMENT

There is a strong correlation between period of gestation at the time of previous PA and the chance of recurrence in the present pregnancy. Some biochemical parameters that may help identify women at high risk of abruption include low plasma-associated placental protein–A in the first trimester, elevated α-feto protein in the second trimester, and abnormal uterine artery waveforms. The use of low-dose aspirin has been found to be beneficial in high-risk women with a history of preeclampsia and its adverse perinatal outcomes such as abruption in a previous pregnancy. For a woman who has had a major PA in the previous pregnancy, surveillance in the present pregnancy should begin at least 6 weeks prior to the period of gestation at which the previous PA occurred [26]. Recent studies have also emphasized close maternal and fetal monitoring at least 6 weeks ahead of previous abruption, as 60% recur around the same gestation period, whereas 40% recur at unrelated gestation [27,39]. Recurrent abruption after an uncomplicated abruption in previous pregnancy is less frequent. Frequent surveillance in a case of previous abruption is based on the hypothesis that a timely identification of abruption in the index pregnancy may have a beneficial outcome; however, there is a lack of prospective studies to validate this assumption. Women at risk of recurrence of abruption need screening for placental function and fetal growth. The presence of hypertension, chronic or gestational, further increases the risk of PA; hence, control of hypertension is mandatory.

TIMING OF DELIVERY

The risk of PA increases with advancing gestation, especially after 37 weeks of gestation. Induction of labor is recommended at 37 weeks of gestation [39]; however, the practice at Parkland Hospital, Texas, USA is to terminate pregnancy at 38 weeks period of gestation if no other complication develops prior to this [43].

CONCLUSION

There is enough evidence to suggest that poor reproductive performance in a woman caused by either hypertension in pregnancy or due to placental abruption is likely to impact future pregnancies, in addition to the presence of either recognized or unrecognized etiology. This is more likely in early-onset preeclampsia and in women with nontoxemic abruption of placenta, as hypertension occurring in the latter half of pregnancy is less likely to recur, therefore decreasing the recurrence of toxemic abruption.

REFERENCES

1. World Health Organization (WHO). *The World Health Report: 2005: Make Every Mother and Child Count*. Geneva, Switzerland: WHO; 2005.
2. Duley L. Maternal mortality associated with hypertensive disorders of pregnancy in Africa, Asia, Latin America and the Caribbean. *Br J Obstet Gynaecol*. 1992;99:547–53.
3. Homer CS, Brown MA, Mangos G, Davis GK. Non-proteinuric pre-eclampsia: A novel risk indicator in women with gestational hypertension. *J Hypertens*. 2008;26:295–302.
4. American College of Obstetricians and Gynecologists (ACOG). Diagnosis and management of preeclampsia and eclampsia. ACOG Practice Bulletin No. 33. *Obstet Gynecol*. 2002;99:159–67.
5. Report of the National High Blood Pressure Education Program Working Group on High Blood Pressure in Pregnancy. *Am J Obstet Gynecol*. 2000;183:S1–22.
6. Auger N, Fraser WD, Schnitzer M, Leduc L, Healy-Profitos J, Paradis G. Recurrent preeclampsia and subsequent cardiovascular risk. *Heart*. 2017;103:235–43.
7. Bramham K, Briley AL, Seed P, Poston L, Shennan AH, Chappell LC. Adverse maternal and perinatal outcomes in women with previous preeclampsia: A prospective study. *Am J Obstet Gynecol*. 2011;204:512.e1–9.
8. Callaway LK, Mamun A, McIntyre HD, Williams GM, Najman JM, Nitert MD, Lawlor DA. Does a history of hypertensive disorders of pregnancy help predict future essential hypertension? Findings from a prospective pregnancy cohort study. *J Hum Hypertens*. 2013;27:309–14.
9. Hjartardottir S, Leifsson BG, Geirsson RT, Steinthorsdottir V. Recurrence of hypertensive disorder in second pregnancy. *Am J Obstet Gynecol*. 2006;194:916–20.
10. Brown MA, Mackenzie C, Dunsmuir W et al. Can we predict recurrence of pre-eclampsia or gestational hypertension? *BJOG*. 2007;114:984–93.
11. Duckitt K, Harrington D. Risk factors for preeclampsia at antenatal booking: Systematic review of controlled studies. *BMJ*. 2005;330: 565.
12. Blumenthal JA, Babyak MA, Sherwood A et al. Effects of the dietary approaches to stop hypertension diet alone and in combination with exercise and caloric restriction on insulin sensitivity and lipids. *Hypertension*. 2010;55:1199–205.
13. Redman CW, Sargent IL. Latest advances in understanding preeclampsia. *Science*. 2005;308:1592–4.
14. Caritis S, Sibai B, Hauth J et al. Low-dose aspirin to prevent preeclampsia in women at high risk. National Institute of Child Health and Human Development Network of Maternal-Fetal Medicine Units. *N Engl J Med*. 1998;338:701–5.

15. Bujold E, Roberge S, Lacasse Y et al. Prevention of preeclampsia and intrauterine growth restriction with aspirin started in early pregnancy: A meta-analysis. *Obstet Gynecol.* 2010;116:402–14.

16. Duley L, Henderson-Smart DJ, Meher S, King JF. Antiplatelet agents for preventing pre-eclampsia and its complications. *Cochrane Database Sys Rev.* Apr 18, 2007;(2):CD004659.

17. American College of Obstetricians and Gynecologists (ACOG). *Antepartum Fetal Surveillance. ACOG Practice Bulletin 9.* Washington, DC: ACOG; 1999.

18. Magee L, Sadeghi S, von Dadelszen P. Prevention and treatment of postpartum hypertension. *Cochrane Database Syst Rev.* Jan 25, 2005;(1):CD004351.

19. Podymow T, August P. Postpartum course of gestational hypertension and preeclampsia. *Hypertens Pregnancy.* 2010;29:294–300.

20. Irgens HU, Reisaeter L, Irgens LM, Lie RT. Long term mortality of mothers and fathers after pre-eclampsia: Population based cohort study. *BMJ.* 2001;323:1213–7.

21. Mongraw-Chaffin ML, Cirillo PM, Cohn BA. Preeclampsia and cardiovascular disease death: Prospective evidence from the child health and development studies cohort. *Hypertension.* 2010;56:166–71.

22. Ray JG, Vermeulen MJ, Schull MJ, Redelmeier DA. Cardiovascular health after maternal placental syndromes (CHAMPS): Population-based retrospective cohort study. *Lancet.* 2005;366:1797–803.

23. Funai EF, Paltiel OB, Malaspina D, Friedlander Y, Deutsch L, Harlap S. Risk factors for pre-eclampsia in nulliparous and parous women: The Jerusalem perinatal study. *Paediatr Perinat Epidemiol.* 2005;19:59–68.

24. Romundstad PR, Magnussen EB, Smith GD, Vatten LJ. Hypertension in pregnancy and later cardiovascular risk: Common antecedents? *Circulation.* 2010;122:579–84.

25. Mosca L, Benjamin EJ, Berra K et al. Effectiveness-based guidelines for the prevention of cardiovascular disease in women—2011 update: A guideline from the American Heart Association. American Heart Association [published erratum appears in *J Am Coll Cardiol.* 2012;59:1663]. *J Am Coll Cardiol.* 2011;57:1404–23.

26. Rasmussen S, Irgens LM, Dalaker K. The effect on the likelihood of further pregnancy of placental abruption and the rate of its recurrence. *Br J Obstet Gynaecol.* 1997;104:1292–5.

27. Rasmussen S, Irgens LM, Dalaker K. Outcome of pregnancies subsequent to placental abruption: A risk assessment. *Acta Obstet Gynecol Scand.* 2000;79:496–501.

28. Raymond EG, Mills JL. Placental abruption: Maternal risk factors and associated fetal conditions. *Acta Obstet Gynecol Scand.* 1993;72:633–9.

29. Ananth CV, Oyelese Y, Srinivas N, Yeo L, Vintzileos AM. Preterm premature rupture of membranes, intrauterine infection and oligohydramnios: Risk factors for placental abruption. *Obstet Gynecol.* 2004;104:71–7.

30. Tikkanen M, Nuutila M, Hiilesmaa V, Paavonen J, Ylikorkala O. Clinical presentation and risk factors of placental abruption. *Acta Obstet Gynecol Scand.* 2006;85:700–5.

31. Tikkanen M, Nuutila M, Hiilesmaa V, Paavonen J, Ylikorkala O. Prepregnancy risk factors for placental abruption. *Acta Obstet Gynecol Scand.* 2006;85:40–4.

32. Ananth CV, Nath CA, Philipp C. The normal anticoagulant system and risk of placental abruption: Protein C, protein S and resistance to activated protein C. *J Matern Fetal Neonatal Med.* 2010;23:1377–83.

33. Deutsch AB, Lynch O, Alio AP, Salihu HM, Spellacy WN. Increased risk of placental abruption in underweight women. *Am J Perinatol.* 2010;27:235–40.

34. Rasmussen S, Irgens LM. Occurrence of placental abruption in relatives. *BJOG.* 2009;116:693–9.

35. Tikkanen M. Etiology, clinical manifestations, and prediction of placental abruption. *Acta Obstet Gynecol Scand.* 2010;89:732–40.

36. Pariente G, Wiznitzer A, Sergienko R, Mazor M, Holcberg G, Sheiner E. Placental abruption: Critical analysis of risk factors and perinatal outcomes. *J Matern Fetal Neonatal Med.* 2010;24:698–702.

37. Kennare R, Heard A, Chan A. Substance use during pregnancy: Risk factors and obstetric and perinatal outcomes in South Australia. *ANZJOG.* 2005;45:220–5.

38. Robertson L, Wu O, Langhorne P et al. Thrombosis: Risk and economic assessment

of thrombophilia screening (TREATS) Study. Thrombophilia in pregnancy: A systematic review. *Br J Haematol.* 2006;132:171–96.

39. Ruiter L, Ravelli ACJ, de Graaf IM et al. Incidence and recurrence rate of placental abruption: A longitudinal linked national cohort study in the Netherlands. *Am J Obstet Gynecol.* 2015;213:573.e1–8.

40. Charles DH, Ness AR, Campbell D, Smith GD, Whitley E, Hall MH. Folic acid supplements in pregnancy and birth outcome: Re-analysis of a large randomised controlled trial and update of Cochrane review. *Paediatr Perinat Epidemiol.* 2005;19:112–24.

41. Rodger MA, Paidas M. Do thrombophilias cause placenta-mediated pregnancy complications? *Semin Thromb Hemost.* 2007;33: 597–603.

42. Gris JC, Chauleur C, Faillie JL et al. Enoxaparin for the secondary prevention of placental vascular complications in women with abruptio placentae: The pilot randomised controlled NOH-AP trial. *Thromb Haemost.* 2010;104:771–9.

43. Williams J, Cunningham F, Leveno K et al. *Williams Obstetrics.* 25th ed. New York, NY: McGraw-Hill Education; 2018.

9

Approach to women with previous rupture of the uterus or an unknown uterine scar in pregnancy

BHARTI JOSHI

INTRODUCTION

Uterine rupture is defined as complete separation of all uterine walls including serosa resulting in extrusion of the fetus with intra-amniotic contents into the peritoneal cavity. If there is disruption of only uterine musculature with intact serosa, then it is called *uterine dehiscence*. The terms *symptomatic* and *asymptomatic* uterine rupture have been used in the literature to differentiate uterine rupture from dehiscence. Uterine rupture, although rare, is a catastrophic complication associated with high fetal-maternal morbidity and mortality [1,2]. It can result in peripartum hysterectomy, hemorrhagic shock, multiorgan dysfunction, and severe neonatal issues. The disastrous outcome is evident in a review by Eden et al., in which almost 95% of women with ruptured uterus required blood transfusion [3]. Maternal mortality was reported up to 12%, and around 40% of women required peripartum hysterectomy [4]. Hypogastric artery ligation along with good suture repair is considered for women desirous of fertility.

INCIDENCE

The incidence of rupture in an unscarred uterus is reported as 1 in 10,000 births, whereas in women with one previous lower segment scar, it is approximately 0.2%–1.5%. Uterine rupture occurs in 4%–9% of women with previous classic or T-shaped incisions [5–8]. Uterine perforation during curetting and hysteroscopy has also been implicated [9]. Various factors associated with uterine rupture are congenital uterine anomaly, scarred uterus, grand multiparity, and obstetrical conditions like macrosomia, malpresentation, uterine dystocia, attempted instrumental delivery, and injudicious labor [10–12]. Over the years, cases of rupture secondary to dystocia and overuse of oxytocin have decreased, and now they occur more in women with a scarred uterus [9,13]. The rising trend of cesareans, overuse of prostaglandins, and attempts of vaginal delivery in previous cesareans are the main causes of uterine rupture [14–16]. The incidence of uterine rupture in women undergoing labor is 3.8–7 per 1000 births [15,17–19]. The wide variation of incidence reported in the literature between developed and developing nations is probably related to the sociodemographic factors, lack of awareness, access to health care, and adequacy of intrapartum care. A large, retrospective study from Nepal over a period of 20 years quoted the incidence of rupture as 0.09%. Most of the women were multiparous with unscarred uterus [20]. Similarly, Ofir et al. reported rupture in 0.035% of deliveries, and only 10% of women had previous uterine scarring [21]. The Netherland study found rupture in unscarred and scarred uterus in 0.7 and 5.1 per 10,000 deliveries, respectively [22]. Antepartum rupture is mainly reported in women with upper segment scar or history of previous myomectomy [23]. To date, no significant difference has been seen in adverse outcomes related to ruptured uterus in laparoscopic versus open myomectomy; however, large studies are needed to validate this finding [24].

Injudicious use of misoprostol leading to uterine rupture has been reported in past years in many case reports [25]. The incidence of rupture in scarred uterus with misoprostol induction is 5.6% [26].

HOW TO COUNSEL WOMEN WITH A HISTORY OF PREVIOUS UTERINE RUPTURE

Prior uterine rupture is not an absolute contraindication for future pregnancy. The majority of women receiving diligent antenatal care have promising outcomes in subsequent pregnancies. Therefore, any woman with prior uterine rupture who is desirous of conception has to be properly counseled and thoroughly evaluated. Detailed history, critical review of previous records, site of rupture, cause of rupture, repair technique, median interval of previous rupture, and postoperative recovery have to be clearly documented. The site of prior rupture and the interconception period have direct correlation with recurrence of rupture in subsequent pregnancy. In the case of prior rupture confined to the lower uterine segment, the repeat risk is 6% in future pregnancy. In the case of upper segment rupture, the risk is very high, up to 32% [27].

MANAGEMENT OF PREGNANCY IN WOMEN WITH A HISTORY OF PREVIOUS UTERINE RUPTURE

There is no clear evidence for a course of action for subsequent pregnancies in women with conservatively managed uterine rupture. The main focus to prevent subsequent rupture is on the mode and timing of delivery. Review of case reports published so far showed that with adequate antenatal care and a planned elective cesarean, pregnancy outcome in women with prior uterine rupture can be optimized. In a review of five pregnancies after uterine rupture by Lim et al., all were delivered by cesarean, and no one had repeat rupture [28]. Out of these five women, four had elective cesarean in the next pregnancy resulting in the birth of healthy newborns. Three of these four women had cesarean between 36 and 37 weeks after receiving steroids and documentation of fetal lung maturity, and one had cesarean at 38 weeks. One patient underwent emergency peripartum hysterectomy at 30 weeks due to placenta percreta. It is evident that if adequate prenatal care is given, then subsequent rupture can be avoided.

One has to individualize the treatment plan based on previous data about the type of scar, at what gestation labor started and rupture occurred (Figure 9.1). As per the literature, elective cesarean should not be planned before labor or 38 weeks in case of prior lower segment rupture [29,30]. If one decides on cesarean at earlier gestation, then it is advisable to document fetal lung maturity and give steroids [1]. In case a woman had a previous classical scar rupture or a history of preterm labor, early cesarean at 34 weeks should be preferably planned and the woman should be admitted 1 week prior to the gestation at which labor began in previous pregnancy [31].

Keefar et al. reported 253 pregnancies in 194 women after uterine rupture. Out of them, 12.8% had repeat rupture, and two women died. It was observed that the risk of rupture was greatest in women with a history of prior classical scar rupture [32]. In another review, 34 women with prior rupture had 46 pregnancies. Out of them, 27 women had repeat caesareans, three delivered vaginally, and 4 had repeat rupture. Findings revealed that among the cesarean group, 16 had one cesarean, 10 had two cesareans, and one woman underwent three cesareans after prior uterine rupture [33]. Rupture was seen at 40 weeks in one with prior lower segment rupture, another had cornual leak at 22 weeks, while upper segment scar of two others gave way at 22 and 36 weeks. It was concluded from this study that conservative management of uterine rupture is determined by various social,

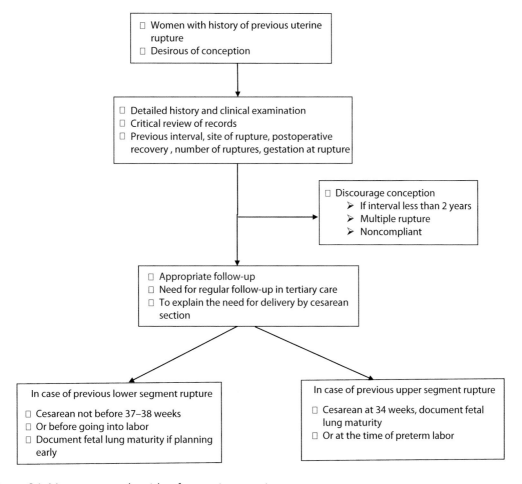

Figure 9.1 Management algorithm for previous uterine rupture.

economic, and religious factors. Repeat risk of rupture can be minimized by proper counseling of the couple, by appropriate record keeping, and by early admission and intervention. There is a case reported where successful cesarean was done in a woman with a history of two occurrences of uterine rupture.

In a 25-year review of uterine rupture and subsequent pregnancy outcomes by Chibber et al., strong emphasis was given to preserve the uterus, especially in women desirous of conception [34,35]. There is no doubt that emergency peripartum hysterectomy is a lifesaving procedure, and the surgical skills and the condition of the patient determine the modality of treatment. The pregnancies in 22 women out of 24 who had uterine repair along with hypogastric artery ligation were reported. All of these women were informed that future delivery would be by the abdominal route, and repeat risk

of rupture was always there [36]. Of them, 73% with previous lower segment rupture had elective cesarean at 37 weeks with no fetal or maternal complications, while 18% with upper uterine segment rupture were delivered at 35 weeks uneventfully. Two noncompliant women with upper segment rupture had repeat rupture followed by catastrophic hemorrhage and mortality. Previous vertical ruptures and shorter intervals between (2 and 5 years) appear to be important risk factors for repeat rupture. Another determinant is period of gestation at prior rupture; the shorter the gestation, the higher the chance of recurrence. Knowing all this helps clinicians begin further counseling and raise the alarm at the slightest indication of rupture [1].

One important decision regarding the timing of delivery in prior uterine rupture comes from a decision analytical model of a theoretical cohort of 100 women. It was observed that elective cesarean at 34 weeks instead of 36 weeks would prevent 3.86 ruptures. This would, in turn, lead to 0.0079 lower maternal deaths but also more cases of cerebral palsy [37]. Delaying delivery up to 36 weeks would result in 0.47 fewer cases of cerebral palsy. Looking at the pros and cons of both, termination at 34 weeks was found to be optimal as it maximizes the neonatal and maternal quality adjusted life-years.

Another group of patients includes those with unknown uterine scar. In these cases, it is difficult to predict and prevent uterine rupture or dehiscence. Out of four women, one can have some kind of morbidity. If there is some evidence from previous records or history that the unknown scar is in the upper segment, then subsequent pregnancy has to be managed like a previous classical scar. Documenting fetal lung maturity at 36–37 weeks and then planning cesarean will result in a good outcome [1]. The risk of uterine rupture in a defective scar is related to its location and thinning with an overall risk of 4%–19% [19]. Therefore, even in a history of previous dilatation and curetting with perforation, one should strictly follow and explain the risk or rupture in subsequent pregnancy.

CONCLUSION

It is evident from the literature that subsequent pregnancy outcome can be optimized in women with prior uterine rupture or dehiscence. A woman with previous rupture of the uterus or unknown uterine scar in pregnancy should be closely monitored and preferably delivered before the onset of labor. One should have a uniform institutional protocol for managing such cases. Because of the rarity of such cases, it is not feasible to conduct prospective trials to develop standardized management policies. It is up to the clinical judgment of the physician to decide about management and timing of delivery in women with a history of uterine rupture in previous pregnancy. An individualistic approach and an informed doctor-patient consensus may improve the likely outcome.

REFERENCES

1. Lim AC, Lau WC, Fung HYM. Pregnancy after uterine rupture: A report of 5 cases and a review of the literature. *Obstet Gynecol Surv.* 2005;60:613–7.

2. Engelson BE, Albrechtsen S, Iversen OE. Peripartum hysterectomy—Incidents and maternal mortality. *Acta Obster Gynecol Scand.* 2001;80:409–12.

3. Eden RD, Parker RT, Gall SG. Rupture of the gravid uterus: A 53 year review. *Obstet Gynecol.* 1986;68:671–4.

4. Lema VM, Ojwang SB, Wanjala SH. Rupture of the gravid uterus: A review. *East Afr Med J.* 1991;68:430–41.

5. Rageth JC, Juzi C, Grossenbacher H. Delivery after previous caesarean: A risk evaluation. Swiss Working Group of Obstetric and Gynecologic Institutions. *Obstet Gynecol.* 1999;93:332–7.

6. Miller DA, Goodwin TM, Gherman RB, Paul RH. Intrapartum rupture of the unscarred uterus. *Obstet Gynecol.* 1997;89(5 Pt 1):671–3.

7. Sweeten KM, Graves WK, Athanassiou A. Spontaneous rupture of the unscarred uterus. *Am J Obstet Hynecol.* 1995;172:1851–6.

8. American College of Obstetricians and Gynecologists. ACOG practice bulletin. Vaginal birth after previous cesarean delivery. No. 5, July 1999 (replaces practice bulletin no. 2, October 1998). Clinical management guidelines for obstetrician-gynecologists. *Int J Gynaecol Obstet.* 1999;66:197–204.

9. Catanzarite VA, Mehalek KE, Wachtel T, Westbrook C. Sonographic diagnosis of traumatic and later recurrent uterine rupture. *Am J Perinatol.* 1996;13:177–80.

10. Farmer RM, Kirschbaum T, Potter D, Strong TH, Medearis AL. Uterine rupture during trial of labor after previous cesarean section. *Am J Obstet Gynecol.* 1991;165(4):996–1001.

11. Miller DA, Diaz FG, Paul RH. Vaginal birth after cesarean: A 10-year experience. *Obstet Gynecol.* 1994;84(2):255–8.

12. Nkemayim DC, Hammadeh ME, Hippach M, Mink D, Schmidt W. Uterine rupture in pregnancy subsequent to previous laparoscopic electromyolysis. Case report and review of the literature. *Arch Gynecol Obstet.* 2000;264(3):154–6.

13. Phelan JP. Uterine rupture. *Clin Obstet Gynecol.* 1990;33:432.

14. Turner MJ. Uterine rupture. *Best Pract Res Clin Obstet Gynaecol.* 2002;16:69–79.

15. Landon MB, Hauth JC, Leveno KJ et al. Maternal and perinatal outcomes associated with a trial of labor after prior cesarean delivery. *N Engl J Med.* 2004;351:2581–9.

16. Khabbaz AY, Usta IM, El-Hajj MI, Abu-Musa A, Seoud M, Nassar AH. Rupture of an unscarred uterus with misoprostol induction: Case report and review of the literature. *J Matern Fetal Med.* 2001;10:141–5.

17. Chauhan SP, Martin JN, Henrichs CE et al. Maternal and perinatal complications with uterine rupture in patients who attempted vaginal birth after cesarean delivery, review of the literature. *Am J Obstet Gynecol.* 2003;189:408–17.

18. Guise JM, McDonagh M, Osterweil P et al. Systematic review of the incidence and consequences of uterine rupture in women with previous caesarean section. *BMJ* 2004;329:1–7.

19. Ramphal SR, Moodley J. Antepartum uterine rupture in previous caesarean sections presenting as advanced extrauterine pregnancies: Lessons learnt. *Eur J Obstet Gynecol Reprod Biol.* 2009;143(1):3–8.

20. Padhye SM. Rupture of the pregnant uterus: A 20 year review. *Kathmandu Univ Med J.* 2005;3:234–8.

21. Ofir K, Sheiner E, Levy A, Katz M, Mazor M. Uterine rupture: Risk factors and pregnancy outcome. *Am J Obstet Gynecol.* 2003;189:1042–6.

22. Zwart JJ, Richters JM, Ory F et al. Uterine rupture in The Netherlands: A nationwide population-based cohort study. *BJOG* 2009;116:1069.

23. Halperin ME, Moore DC, Hannah WJ. Classical versus low-segment transverse section: Maternal complications and outcome of subsequent pregnancies. *Br J Obstet Gynaecol.* 1988;95:990–6.

24. Parker WH, Lacampo K, Long T. Uterine rupture after laparoscopic removal of a pedunculated myoma. *J Minim Invasive Gynecol.* 2007;14:362–4.

25. Khabbax AY, Usta IM, El-Hajj MI, Abu-Musa A, Seoud M, Nassar AH. Rupture of an unscarred uterus with misoprostol induction: Case report and review of literature. *J Maternal Fetal Med.* 2001;10:141–5.

26. Plaut MM, Schwartz ML, Lubarsky SL. Uterine rupture associated with the use of misoprostol in the gravid patient with a previous caesarean section. *Am J Obstet Gyncecol.* 1999;180:1535–42.

27. Ritchie EH. Pregnancy after rupture of the pregnant uterus. A report of 36 pregnancies and a study of cases reported since 1932. *J Obstet Gynecol Br Common.* 1971;78:642–8.

28. Lim AC, Kwee A, Bruinse HW. *Pregnancy after uterine rupture: A report of 5 cases and a review of the literature. Obstet Gynecol Surv.* 2005;60(9):613–7.

29. Graziosi GCM, Bakker CM, Brouwers HA et al. [Elective cesarean section is preferred after the completion of a minimum of 38 weeks of pregnancy]. *Ned Tijdschr Geneesk.* 1998;142:2300–3.

30. Wax JR, Herson V, Carignon E et al. Contribution of elective delivery to severe respiratory distress at term. *Am J Perinatol.* 2002;19:81–6.

31. Fox NS, Gerber RS, Mourad M, Saltzman DH, Klauser CK, Gupta S, Rebarber A. Pregnancy outcomes in patients with prior uterine rupture or dehiscence. *Obstet Gynecol.* 2014;123(4):785–9.

32. Keefer FJ, Walss-Rodriguez R. Successful pregnancy following repair of a ruptured uterus. *W V Med J.* 1975;71:316–9.

33. Onyemeh AU, Twomey D. The consecutive management of uterine rupture. *Trop J Obstet Gynaecol.* 1988;1:80–1.

34. Akhtar N, Parveen T, Sayee S, Begum F. Rupture of primigravid uterus and recurrent rupture a case report. *BSMMU J.* 2013;6(2):168–71.

35. Chibber R, El-Saleh E, Al Fadhli R, Al Jassar W, Al Harm J. Uterine rupture and subsequent pregnancy outcome—How safe is it? A 25-year study. *J Matern Fetal Neonatal Med.* 2010;23(5):421–4.

36. Al Sakka M, Dawdah W, Al Hassan S. Case series of uterine rupture and subsequent pregnancy outcome. *Int J Fertil.* 1999;44:293–300.

37. Frank ZC, Lee VR, Caughey AB. Timing of delivery in women with prior uterine rupture: A decision analysis. *J Matern Fetal Neonatal Med.* Apr 15, 2019:1–7. doi: 10.1080/14767058.2019.1602825.

Approach to women with previous intrapartum stillbirth

BHARTI SHARMA

BACKGROUND AND BURDEN OF STILLBIRTHS

Globally around 2.6 million stillbirths occur per year; half of them (1.2 million) are intrapartum stillbirths, and 98% of this burden is shared by low-middle-income countries [1,2]. Most of these intrapartum stillbirths are attributed to the complications arising during labor and delivery of the fetus, which include prolonged or obstructed labor, umbilical cord prolapse, birth trauma, shoulder dystocia, malpresentation, and birth asphyxia. The proportion of intrapartum stillbirths directly indicates the quality of obstetric care provided to a woman during childbirth and neonatal care at birth. Worldwide, 45 million births, that is, 34% of total births, take place without a skilled birth attendant, especially in low- to middle-income countries [3–5].

DEFINITION

Stillbirth is defined as a baby born with no sign of life after 20 weeks of gestation or birth weight of more than 500 grams. As per the World Health Organization (WHO), fetal death at or after 28 weeks or birth weight of 1000 grams is considered as a stillbirth. Stillbirth is further divided into antepartum and intrapartum depending on the time of fetal death. Intrapartum stillbirth is a death that occurs after the onset of labor and before birth.

CLASSIFICATION FOR CAUSE OF DEATH

There are various classification systems to classify stillbirth, and recently, the WHO recommended a newer classification system, i.e., *International Classification of Diseases, Tenth Revision– Perinatal Mortality (ICD-PM)* [6]. The *ICD-PM* classification system is a multilayered approach to classify stillbirth according to the time of death and maternal and fetal causes separately. Tables 10.1 and 10.2 show the intrapartum stillbirth part of *ICD-PM*. Classification is made with seven subgroups and associated maternal conditions at the time of stillbirth. Delivery time is the best time to evaluate the mother as well as the fetus to reach the actual cause, assessing associated factors that lead to fetal demise. Knowing the actual cause of fetal death not only helps the clinician to manage the woman in her subsequent pregnancies but also helps in counseling, providing bereavement support, and planning preventive strategies. Intrapartum stillbirth deaths are always assumed to be attributed to suboptimal care, negligence, or some intrapartum complications, which is not

Table 10.1 Classification *International Classification of Diseases, Tenth Revision–Perinatal Mortality (ICD-PM)*—Intrapartum Stillbirths

Intrapartum stillbirth—Fetal cause	
Intrapartum death	**ICD-10 coding**
I1 *Congenital malformations*, deformations and chromosomal abnormalities	Q00–Q99
I2 *Birth trauma*	P10–P15
I3 *Acute intrapartum event*	P20.1, P20.9 (intrauterine hypoxia)
I4 *Infection*	P35, P37, P39, A50
I5 *Other specified intrapartum disorder* (fetal blood loss, intracranial nontraumatic hemorrhage, hemolytic disease of fetus and newborn, hydrops fetalis, others)	P50, P52, P55, P56, P60, P61, P70, P96, Misc.
I6 *Disorder related to fetal growth* (slow fetal growth and fetal malnutrition, disorder related to short gestation and low birth weight and long gestation and high birth weight)	P05, P07, P08
I7 *Unspecified cause*	P95

Source: World Health Organization (WHO). *The WHO Application of ICD-10 to Deaths during the Perinatal Period: ICD-PM.* Geneva, Switzerland: WHO; 2016.

always true, especially in resource-constrained settings. That is why it is important to evaluate the maternal condition as well as fetus completely (Table 10.3). For example, intrapartum stillbirths have been reported in women with autoimmune thrombocytopenia due to sudden intracranial bleed (fetal thrombocytopenia) during labor, but to confirm the diagnosis, complete evaluation of both mother and fetus is required, i.e., maternal autoimmune workup, fetal cord blood for platelet count, and fetal magnetic resonance imaging, or autopsy to confirm intracranial bleed. As per *ICD-PM* classification, this stillbirth would be classified as I3—acute intrapartum event and maternal condition, M4—medical disorder of mother. This is why autopsy and placental examination should be offered to all mothers, to be performed after informed consent.

Table 10.2 Maternal condition associated at the time of fetal death

Maternal condition associated with fetal death	Common conditions	*International Classification of Diseases, Tenth Revision (ICD-10)* coding
M1 Complications of placenta, cord, and membranes	Abruption, placenta previa	P02
M2 Maternal complications of pregnancy	Premature rupture of membranes, oligohydramnios, multiple pregnancy	P01
M3 Other complications of labor and delivery	Malpresentation (breech), instrumental delivery complications	P03
M4 Maternal medical and surgical conditions	Hypertensive diseases of pregnancy (preeclampsia, gestational hypertension, eclampsia), diabetes, anemia, infections	P00
M5 No maternal condition (healthy mother)		

Source: World Health Organization (WHO). *The WHO Application of ICD-10 to Deaths during the Perinatal Period: ICD-PM.* Geneva, Switzerland: WHO; 2016.

Table 10.3 Maternal and fetal evaluation at the time of fetal death

Maternal evaluation	Fetal evaluation after birth
Review the history (presenting symptoms, obstetric history, past history) again and look for the risk factors	External examination of fetus, placenta and cord to look for any externally visible birth defects or any birth trauma
Investigations in all cases	**Investigations**
• Complete blood count	• Cord blood ABG, hemogram, platelet count
• Biochemistry including bile salts	• Infantogram/x-ray
• Coagulation profile	• Autopsy including histopathologic examination
• Blood group and antibody titers	• Fetal and placental microbiology
• Hemoglobin electrophoresis	
• Random blood glucose	
• Glycosylated hemoglobin	
• Thyroid function	
• Kleihauer-Betke test	
• Serology for viral screen, syphilis, tropical infection	
In selected cases	**In selected cases**
• Maternal bacteriology—maternal fever, flu-like symptoms	• Fetal and placental tissue for karyotype (selected cases)
• Abnormal liquor, prolonged leaking PV	
• Maternal thrombophilia screen	
• Anti-red cell antibody serology	
• Maternal anti-Ro and anti-La antibodies	
• Maternal alloimmune antiplatelet antibodies	
• Parental karyotype	
• Fetal unbalanced translocation	
• Other fetal aneuploidy	
• Fetal abnormality on autopsy	
• Previous unexplained stillbirth	

Abbreviations: ABG, arterial blood gas; PV, per vaginum.

Approach to women with previous intrapartum stillbirth (Table 10.4)

PRECONCEPTION CARE

Women with previous stillbirths are at a higher risk of adverse pregnancy outcomes such as preterm labor, abruption, low birth weight, and stillbirth in subsequent pregnancies as compared to women with live births. Previous stillbirth is an important risk factor, and risk of recurrence depends on the cause of death. So it is crucial to assign the cause of a previous stillbirth to plan care in subsequent pregnancy. When such a woman comes for preconception care, it is important to examine the woman and review here previous obstetric history, past history, and available documents. Review the autopsy and placental examination report and assign the most probable cause for fetal death if not assigned earlier. Women with modifiable risk factors like diabetes, hypertension, smoking, obesity, and so on, should be advised to optimize their health status before planning their next pregnancy. Stillbirths attributed to intrapartum complications like birth trauma and acute intrapartum events should be addressed of better outcomes in subsequent pregnancies with the availability of comprehensive emergency obstetric care and skilled birth attendants. In unexplained or unspecified death, it has been recommended that women be managed as presumed placental cause [7,8].

CARE DURING SUBSEQUENT PREGNANCY

The women who had a previous intrapartum stillbirth should be supervised at a tertiary care center or should seek care from experts or skilled community practitioners experienced in the management of such subsequent pregnancies. These mothers need compassionate

Table 10.4 Approach to women with previous intrapartum stillbirth [7–9]

Preconception care
- Detailed history and clinical examination
- Review of records (autopsy findings, placental examination report, karyotype)
- Assign the cause for previous intrapartum loss
- Rule out underlying chronic diseases: Hypertension, diabetes mellitus, thyroid disorders
- Folic acid supplementation
- Reassurance and psychosocial support to woman and her family

During subsequent pregnancy at booking

First trimester
- Ultrasound—Confirmation of pregnancy and dating
- Folic acid to continue, low-dose aspirin in indicated cases
- Aneuploidy screening (11–13 weeks)
- Glucose tolerance test, thyroid function
- Reassurance and psychosocial support to woman and her family

Second trimester
- Level II ultrasound (cervical length monitoring in cases of previous history of cervical incompetence or prematurity-related loss)
- Aneuploidy screening
- Uterine artery Doppler (optional)
- Reassurance and psychosocial support to woman and her family

Third trimester
- Glucose tolerance test (third trimester/24–28 weeks)
- Ultrasound for serial growth monitoring (28 weeks onward, every 2 weeks)
- Daily fetal movement count (28 weeks)
- Nonstress test (optional)
- Reassurance and psychosocial support to woman and her family

Delivery
- Induction at 39 weeks or earlier if indicated but not before 37 weeks of gestation

Mode of delivery
- Vaginal delivery preferably after informed consent of a woman
- Cesarean delivery where induction is contraindicated

care along with medical treatment that will also help in relieving their anxiety of recurrence [7–9].

MEDICAL INTERVENTION DURING PREGNANCY

Intrapartum stillbirths attributed to suboptimal care, birth trauma, or cord prolapse are nonrecurrent conditions, and these mothers do not require any specific medical intervention. But cases where there is evidence of placental insufficiency or fetal growth restrictions or preeclampsia may benefit from low-dose aspirin. Low-dose aspirin should be initiated before 16 weeks of gestation and continued until delivery. Women who had birth defect–related intrapartum loss need genetic counseling and preconception folic acid intake in cases of neural tube defects. So for each case, the plan should be individualized depending on the cause of the previous stillbirth [7–9].

PRENATAL INVESTIGATION

Routine prenatal investigation that includes hemogram, infection screen (human immunodeficiency virus, HBsAg, hepatitis C virus, VDRL), blood group, hemoglobin electrophoresis, thyroid function test, and glucose tolerance test (GTT) should be done at the time of booking [7–9]. In addition, aneuploidy screening (dual screening, ultrasound for nuchal thickness [NT] and nasal bone, quadruple screening) can also be done as per recommendations. The highest recurrence of stillbirth has been seen in cases that are mediated by placental growth factors and prematurity. There are some biochemical parameters like low plasma-associated placental protein–A (PAPP-A) value and uterine artery Doppler abnormalities that are found to be associated with stillbirths [10,11]. But these tests are not recommended routinely due to poor predictive value, as there is already a high risk of recurrence in cases of previous stillbirths.

ANTEPARTUM SURVEILLANCE

As such, there are limited data to guide how frequently these women should be seen for prenatal checkups, but they definitely require more vigilant monitoring and psychological support during their pregnancy. It has been found in various studies that women with previous stillbirths are at an increased risk of having low birth weight babies; therefore, along with frequent prenatal visits, they need additional ultrasounds for serial growth monitoring to check for fetal growth retardation. The American College of Obstetricians and Gynecologists (ACOG) recommends starting antepartum testing at 32–34 weeks, whereas the Society of Obstetricians and Gynaecologists of Canada (SOGC) suggests starting at 28 weeks or earlier with consideration given to the gestation age of the previous loss [8,9]. Fetal biometry should be performed at 2-week intervals, although there are no data available in support of performing a routine biophysical profile at every visit. As such, there is no clear evidence as to whether increasing monitoring and more frequent ultrasounds will help these women or lead to more anxiety.

ROLE OF DAILY FETAL MOVEMENT COUNT

It is a routine practice to offer daily fetal movement count to all pregnant women after 28 weeks of gestation, and it is strictly emphasized to women with previous stillbirth. As per Cochrane review (2015), there is no evidence to support the impact of fetal movement count in the reduction of perinatal mortality [12,13]. However, Tveit et al. reported a reduction in stillbirths by educating the women and using fetal movement count as a "self-screening" test and report to the health-care provider on time [14].

TIMING OF DELIVERY

For intrapartum stillbirth, there is no recommendation for the timing of delivery, but it is stressful to both the patient as well as care provider to decide the delivery time. The care provider has to reassure the woman and keep the risk of iatrogenic prematurity and fetal well-being in mind. Different regions offer induction from early term (37 weeks) to term (39 weeks), but to date, there is no uniform consensus. Ideally, each case should be individualized, considering gestation of previous stillbirths, circumstances during previous delivery, and emotional state of the mother, before planning induction before 39 weeks. The woman and her family should be clearly informed about the neonatal complications associated with induction of labor before 39 weeks, such as transient tachypnea of the newborn, need for neonatal intensive care unit admission, and remote chances of cerebral palsy.

MODE OF DELIVERY

There are no data or evidence to support the mode of delivery with respect to perinatal mortality, morbidity, or maternal psychological morbidity. But a woman who had a previous intrapartum stillbirth will definitely opt for planned cesarean section. The decision for mode of delivery should be a joint decision of the woman and her care provider. The associated advantages and disadvantages of both cesarean and vaginal delivery should be explained in detail to the woman [7–9].

BEREAVEMENT CARE AND PSYCHOSOCIAL SUPPORT

Stillbirth is a devastating event that not only affects the woman but their families and society as well. The psychological impact in the form of anxiety, depression, complicated grief, coping issues, and posttraumatic stress continue beyond the postpartum period. These women need emotional and psychosocial support throughout their pregnancy. But it has been reported in a number of studies that the psychosocial needs are not adequately addressed; care providers tend to emphasize the prevention of medical complications over emotional support [15,16].

CONCLUSION

Women with previous intrapartum stillbirths need individualized consistent medical and psychosocial care since the time of stillbirth through a subsequent pregnancy and beyond. Each case has to be individualized according to the cause of stillbirth, current pregnancy complications, and emotional well-being. The decision of time and mode of delivery should be an informed choice and the joint decision of both the woman and her care provider on the basis of available evidence.

REFERENCES

1. Lawn JE, Yakoob MY, Haws RA, Soomro T, Darmstadt GL, Bhutta ZA. 3.2 million stillbirths: Epidemiology and overview of the evidence review. *BMC Pregnancy Childbirth.* 2009;9(Suppl 1):S2.
2. Lawn J, Shibuya K, Stein C. No cry at birth: Global estimates of intrapartum stillbirths and intrapartum-related neonatal deaths. *Bull World Health Organ.* 2005;83(6):409–17.
3. World Health Organization (WHO). *Neonatal and Perinatal Mortality. Country, Regional and Global Estimates.* Geneva, Switzerland: WHO; 2006.
4. Skill Birth Attendants. https://www.who.int/gho/maternal_health/skilled_care/skilled_birth_attendance_text/en/
5. Darmstadt GL, Lee AC, Cousens S et al. 60 Million non-facility births: Who can deliver in community settings to reduce intrapartum-related deaths? *Int J Gynaecol Obstet.* 2009;107(Suppl 1):S89–112.
6. World Health Organization (WHO). The WHO Application of ICD-10 to Deaths during the Perinatal Period: ICD-PM. Geneva, Switzerland: WHO; 2016.
7. Ladhani NN, Fockler ME, Stephens L, Barrett JF, Heazell AE. No. 369—Management of pregnancy subsequent to stillbirth. *J Obstet Gynaecol Canada.* 2018;40(12):1669–83.
8. Royal College of Obstetricians and Gynaecologists (RCOG). Late Intrauterine Fetal Death and Stillbirth. No. 55 Green-top guidelines. London, UK: RCOG; 2010.
9. American College of Obstetricians and Gynecologists. ACOG Practice Bulletin No. 102: Management of stillbirth. *Obstet Gynecol.* 2009;113(3):748–61.
10. Mastrodima S, Akolekar R, Yerlikaya G, Tzelepis T, Nicolaides KH. Prediction of stillbirth from biochemical and biophysical markers at 11–13 weeks. *Ultrasound Obstet Gynecol.* 2016;48:613–7.
11. Kumar M, Singh S, Sharma K, Singh R, Ravi V, Bhattacharya J. Adverse fetal outcome: Is first trimester ultrasound and Doppler better predictor than biomarkers? *J Matern Fetal Neonatal Med.* Jun 18, 2017;30(12):1410–6.
12. Mangesi L, Hofmeyr GJ, Smith V, Smyth RM. Fetal movement counting for assessment of fetal wellbeing. *Cochrane Database of Syst Rev.* 2015;(10).
13. Winje BA, Wojcieszek AM, Gonzalez-Angulo LY et al. Interventions to enhance maternal awareness of decreased fetal movement: A systematic review. *BJOG* 2016;123:886–98.
14. Tveit JV, Saastad E, Stray-Pedersen B et al. Reduction of late stillbirth with the introduction of fetal movement information and guidelines—A clinical quality improvement. *BMC Pregnancy Childbirth.* 2009;9(1):32.
15. Caelli K, Downie J, Letendre A. Parents' experiences of midwife-managed care following the loss of a baby in a previous pregnancy. *J Adv Nurs.* 2002;39:127–36.
16. Cote-Arsenault D, Schwartz K, Krowchuk H, McCoy TP. Evidence-based intervention with women pregnant after perinatal loss. *MCN Am J Matern Child Nurs.* 2014;39:177–86; quiz 87–8.

11

Management of pregnancy with a history of shoulder dystocia and difficult delivery

SEEMA CHOPRA

INTRODUCTION

Shoulder dystocia is defined as the inability to deliver the shoulders once the fetal head has delivered, even with gentle traction in a downward direction. It is reported in 0.2%–3% of deliveries, and the main culprits of this major obstetric emergency usually cited are fetal macrosomia and maternal diabetes [1,2]. Another proposed definition of dystocia given in the literature is when additional maneuvers are required to deliver the shoulders during vaginal birth of a fetus after delivery of the fetal head, which is not relieved by downward traction on the fetal head. Objectively, one can make the diagnosis when the head and body delivery interval is prolonged to more than 60 seconds [3].

Typically, this occurs when the pubic symphysis obstructs the further descent of the anterior shoulder once the head has delivered, sometimes even the posterior shoulder can get impacted on the sacral promontory in the maternal pelvis. Vaginal birth associated with this complication results in an increase in maternal morbidity, such as risk of postpartum hemorrhage (11%) and a number of perineal injuries (3.6%). Although major fetal injuries do not occur in a large number of such cases, neonatal injuries such as injuries to the brachial plexus and bony injuries such as fracture of the clavicle and humerus sometimes result from difficult delivery. There are usually no long-term complications secondary to these events [4]. Diaphragmatic palsy, facial nerve, and sympathetic nerve plexus injury leading to Horner syndrome occasionally occur along with trauma to the brachial plexus [5]. Rarely, there are reports of spiral fracture of the forearm bones and paresis laryngeal nerve in the fetus [6,7].

In 2.3%–16% of deliveries complicated by shoulder dystocia, brachial plexus injury (BPI) of the fetus results. Unfortunately, in around 10% of such cases, the outcome is worse in the form of permanent neurologic damage, while the majority do not lead to any long-term disability [8]. It is reported to occur in 0.43 per 1000 live births in the United Kingdom and Ireland and is reported to be the basis of most common medicolegal complaints related to shoulder dystocia. It is the third most common cause of litigation due to obstetric complication in the United Kingdom. The substandard care was reported to be the cause in 46% of these injuries by the National Health Service Litigation Authority (NHSLA) [9]. At the same time, it was also emphasized that excess traction during a difficult vaginal birth by health-care professionals may not be the only causative factor, as there is strong evidence to suggest the contribution of maternal propulsive forces during labor [10].

There are two main issues pertaining to shoulder dystocia. First, it is not easily predictable in spite of certain recognized risk factors such as increasing parity and birth weight, maternal weight gain during pregnancy, prior macrosomic baby, and maternal diabetes. Second, prevention of dystocia is not possible with elective labor induction in suspected fetal macrosomia [1].

Although various antepartum and risk factors for intrapartum events can lead to shoulder dystocia, the positive predictive value of these factors either alone or in combination is not high, as they can predict only 16% of such cases that result in neonatal morbidity [11]. Even a high estimated fetal weight cannot predict in which case shoulder dystocia will complicate vaginal delivery because an accurate estimation of fetal anthropometry is not easy and also because most of live borns weighing 4500 g deliver uneventfully [12]. On the contrary, in infants less than 4000 g, nearly half of births are complicated by shoulder dystocia [13]. When comparing same birth weight infants of diabetic mothers with those of nondiabetic mothers, the risk increases two- to fourfold in the former [11]. Evaluating the cases of shoulder dystocia in relation to birth weight and maternal diabetes, most cases occur in normal-sized infants born to nondiabetic women; as could be seen in a study of 221, more than 50% of the infants had a birth weight below 4000 g, and 80% of mothers were not diabetic [14]. Similarly, only half of such cases could be predicted with certainty in either maternal diabetes or suspected macrosomic fetuses. The literature suggests that the presence of obstetric risk factors, alone or in combination, such as excessive prepregnancy weight or gestational weight gain, instrumental vaginal delivery, labor induction or augmentation with oxytocin, labor analgesia, and complication of second stage of labor, either precipitated or prolonged, cannot predict which cases will have shoulder dystocia [15]. The risk of recurrent shoulder dystocia increases in subsequent vaginal deliveries [16].

RISK FACTORS

Diabetes mellitus

As the birth weight increases in infants of diabetic women, it translates into a very high likelihood of shoulder dystocia compared to the nondiabetic cohort [17]. The fetal biometry in diabetic mothers (IDMs) differs from the infants of nondiabetic women, especially the chest-to-head and shoulder-to-head ratios that are higher in the former, which specifically increases the risk of dystocia not related to estimated fetal weight and birth weight of less than 4000 g [18]. A biochemical marker of significance is one out-of-range glucose level in a 75 g 2-hour glucose tolerance test, which is a risk factor for macrosomia and shoulder dystocia, thereby causing adverse pregnancy outcome [19].

Previous shoulder dystocia

Shoulder dystocia in prior delivery is a risk factor for recurrence. Although the literature reports the incidence of recurrence to be at least 10% with a range of 1%–16.7% in different studies, recurrence risks ranging from 1% to 25% have been reported in retrospective studies [13,16,20]. However, it is difficult to ascertain the actual risk because seldom is an attempt at labor given with prior history of complicated delivery or neonatal birth injury. It is recommended to evaluate the proposed risk factors in patients with prior shoulder dystocia and plan delivery accordingly. The available history from the clinical notes, plans for future childbearing, and preferred mode of delivery in the present pregnancy should be reviewed before making a final decision. It is imperative to discuss the associated risks and likely benefits of cesarean delivery with the patient, even though the literature does not recommend elective cesarean section for the prevention of dystocia in the present pregnancy.

Fetal macrosomia as a risk factor for shoulder dystocia and modifiable factors for prevention of macrosomia

As most stated risk factors are weakly predictive of morbidity from shoulder dystocia, there are no set guidelines on the basis of clinical scenarios, as no identifiable risk factors can be found in almost half of deliveries complicated by shoulder dystocia [33]. Fetal macrosomia is considered to be one of the risk factors that can lead to shoulder dystocia. It is classified as either the absolute birth weight more than 4000 g, 4500 g, or 5000 g, or according to nomograms in terms of percentile of more than

90th, 95th, or 97th percentile, respectively, for that gestational age. When there is a prior history of delivery of an infant weighing more than 4500 g, the recurrence rate of shoulder dystocia is reported to be as high as 32% compared to a minuscule risk of 0.3% with delivery of a normal birth weight infant the first time. Taking into account maternal factors predisposing to this complication, prepregnancy weight and gain during pregnancy, gestational age at delivery, and alteration in carbohydrate metabolism are considered potentially modifiable predictors of birth weight. Out of these predisposing factors, altered glucose metabolism is considered to be the most significant one, which is also most amenable to intervention. The U.S. Preventive Services Task Force and the National Institutes of Health concluded that treatment of gestational diabetes can reduce the probability of high birth weight of fetus (relative risk [RR] 0.50%, 95% confidence interval [CI] 0.35–0.71) and, in turn, shoulder dystocia (RR 0.42%, 95% CI 0.23–0.77) [34]. The incidence of birth weight above the 95th percentile is up to 35% in diabetic mothers. The Hyperglycemia and Adverse Pregnancy Outcome (HAPO) study showed a significant progressive correlation between maternal glucose levels during 24–32 weeks' gestational age with increased antepartum complications such as preeclampsia as well as adverse perinatal outcomes such as birth weight greater than the 90th percentile, which further adds to the risk of shoulder dystocia and birth injury, need for cesarean birth, and increased risk of neonatal hypoglycemia [19]. Various metabolic factors in addition to good but not stringent glycemic control in women with pregestational diabetes can be responsible for fetal macrosomia; thus, the frequency of macrosomia and shoulder dystocia in this population may not decrease significantly [35].

CAN SHOULDER DYSTOCIA BE PREDICTED?

It is not possible to identify the risk factor in nearly 50% of deliveries complicated by shoulder dystocia, and even when present, this complication can be predicted in less than 10% of cases [15]. There are many factors that may help predict shoulder dystocia recurrence if vaginal delivery is allowed in subsequent pregnancy. The study by Moore et al. shows an increasing incidence in the index pregnancy when the expected birth weight is 3500 g or higher. The risk increases proportionately with vacuum extraction, as instrumental delivery sometimes is an indirect indicator of cephalopelvic disproportion that can recur in the subsequent pregnancy and thus predispose to recurrent shoulder dystocia [20]. However, the risk was not increased with forceps delivery, maternal body mass index (BMI), and gestational weight gain. In addition, the authors did not find a significant association between risk of recurrent shoulder dystocia in the presence of gestational diabetes or the need for instrumental delivery in the subsequent pregnancy. This may be because in women with gestational diabetes mellitus (GDM) or who had severe shoulder dystocia in index pregnancy, there are 50% increased chances of cesarean delivery in subsequent pregnancies; thus, the actual risk of recurrent dystocia cannot be estimated if all such cases were allowed vaginal delivery. The association of shoulder dystocia with fetal macrosomia is quite predictable, which has a significant 13.8% risk of shoulder dystocia in subsequent vaginal delivery [21].

In women with diabetes, considering only the estimated birth weight, a decision-analysis model showed that using a weight greater than 4500 g as a cutoff for mode of delivery, in order to prevent a single complication of permanent neurological damage caused by intrapartum shoulder dystocia, 443 women with this risk factor will have to undergo cesarean birth [22]. In nondiabetic women, a significantly high number, i.e., 3695 cesarean deliveries, would need to be performed to achieve the same result. Hence, in nondiabetic women, a threshold weight of 5000 g for cesarean delivery is estimated to prevent at least 20% of cases of shoulder dystocia without increasing the total cesarean rate, as at this birth weight 50%–60% of infants are delivered abdominally [23]. It is possible to prevent long-term injury to the brachial plexus in shoulder dystocia by applying an algorithm of management of shoulder dystocia, taking into consideration the birth weight as a risk factor.

Prolonged second stage as predictor of shoulder dystocia

A prolonged second stage during vaginal birth in diabetic women with estimated fetal weight of 4000–4500 g or 5000 g in nondiabetic mothers and therefore an increased incidence of operative vaginal delivery can predispose these women to the risk of shoulder dystocia. The principle of intrapartum cesarean delivery over and above low pelvic or outlet operative vaginal delivery in order to prevent morbidity from shoulder dystocia should be applied in such situations [3]. No specific abnormalities of the second stage of labor, such as either prolonged labor or precipitate labor, could predict the occurrence of shoulder dystocia or neonatal injury with accuracy. Results of the comparison of 276 consecutive cases of shoulder dystocia with 600 matched controls showed similar outcomes, even in diabetic women or with suspected fetal macrosomia. It is important for the attending clinicians to be fully aware of predisposing risk factors for shoulder dystocia in labor, and they should anticipate and be prepared to manage it if it occurs [36].

In pregnant women with pregestational diabetes, associated maternal and perinatal risks guide the timing and mode of delivery and not the risk of shoulder dystocia alone. The author believes that based on results of the two trials, one can discuss the pros and cons of elective induction at 39 weeks of gestation in the mother as well as the increased risk of respiratory distress and need for intensive care in the neonate compared to anticipated reduction in shoulder dystocia in women who have gestational diabetes and estimated birth weight of 4000–4500 g. Similar observations were documented in a systematic review including this trial and four observational studies supporting that with active intervention (induction, cesarean delivery), the rates of macrosomia and related complications were reduced. There was heterogeneity in study designs, so conclusions regarding selection criteria of pregnancies requiring elective induction versus cesarean delivery versus expectant management and at what gestational age for the intervention are lacking [37].

PREVENTION OF SHOULDER DYSTOCIA

Planned induction of labor before term in suspected fetal macrosomia—Is it helpful?

Retrospective cohort studies have not shown consistent better outcomes of elective induction of labor as a risk reduction strategy for decreasing the incidence of shoulder dystocia in cases of suspected fetal macrosomia or diabetic women. The American College of Obstetricians and Gynecologists (ACOG) [2] and Cochrane systematic review [24] also do not recommend elective labor induction in suspected large for dates fetus irrespective of the gestational age, as there is a lack of sufficient data supporting a perceived benefit of intervention versus expectant management of pregnancy, awaiting spontaneous labor unless induction is medically indicated [25,26]. Further studies on induction should clarify the optimal gestational age for planning termination and should also focus on tools to diagnose macrosomia for providing better and more accurate diagnosis in order to decrease the incidence of shoulder dystocia [24].

Suspected fetal macrosomia and role of elective cesarean section to prevent shoulder dystocia

Most experts opine that planned cesarean delivery is appropriate in the presence of documented risk factors, thereby reducing the incidence of long-term morbidity associated with this potential complication when vaginal delivery is allowed. Although this will prevent some shoulder dystocias and their associated complications, it has been proven in the literature that the predictive value of various associated risk factors is low, including those factors that actually lead to neonatal complications, and therefore, prevention is not always successful [27]. It is known that dystocia does not occur in a large majority of cases of suspected fetal macrosomia who deliver vaginally. Therefore, conducting cesarean delivery of all such fetuses in order to lower the incidence of this complication will lead to unacceptable high rates of abdominal delivery. Taking into consideration the predictability of sonographic assessment of 4500 g or higher birth weight for diagnosing macrosomia and its effect on elective cesarean delivery as a preventive measure, the analysis of two such reports stated that based on this factor alone, 3695 prophylactic cesarean deliveries were helpful in preventing one neonatal permanent BPI, with an added cost of $8.7 million for each such outcome [22].

ROLE OF OBSTETRICIAN IN MANAGING SHOULDER DYSTOCIA

A literature search shows scant scientific data that favor the universal practice of episiotomy in all cases of shoulder dystocia [28] (Figure 11.1). Regarding the role of the obstetrician in this challenging situation, the literature does not favor one maneuver over another for managing this complication. It is well documented in the trials that the dreaded complication of neonatal BPI may result from any maneuver in carrying out shoulder disimpaction and thus causing stretch on the nerves of the brachial plexus [2]. There are various maneuvers that can be of help when shoulder dystocia occurs at the time of delivery. The first maneuver that should be put into practice is the McRoberts maneuver as it is quite simple and entails hyperflexion of the maternal thighs onto her abdomen. It is successful in a significant number of cases, and the shoulders can usually be disimpacted without much trauma to the infant as well as the parturient [29]. Simultaneously, suprapubic pressure is given by the assistant with the palm so as to abduct and rotate the anterior shoulder in a downward and lateral direction that resolves its impaction. Use of fundal pressure worsens the shoulder impaction, and uterine rupture may occur due to undue force; therefore, this should not be employed at any time in these cases [12]. If still not successful, one can attempt delivery of the posterior arm instead of the anterior arm, which has been shown to be highly successful in alleviating dystocia and achieving vaginal delivery [30]. In almost all such cases, the complications of shoulder dystocia can be resolved within a time frame of less than 5 minutes with the help of these maneuvers [29].

Occasionally, the shoulders are not delivered with these simple maneuvers if there is a severe degree of shoulder dystocia. In such rare and difficult situations, the Zavanelli maneuver is described, which entails cephalic replacement into the vagina manually followed by cesarean delivery. This maneuver is associated with significant fetal morbidity and mortality and maternal morbidity but may have to be used to relieve catastrophic cases of shoulder dystocia [31]. Another less practiced procedure is abdominal rescue, which

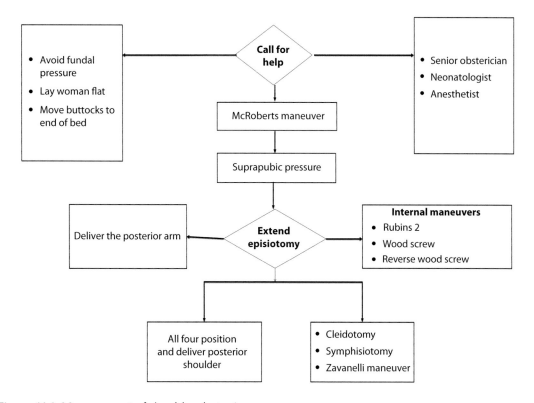

Figure 11.1 Management of shoulder dystocia.

involves hysterotomy for dislodging the anterior shoulder manually through the uterine incision followed by vaginal delivery [32]. Sometimes the obstetrician delivering the fetus causes a fracture of the fetal clavicle intentionally by hooking it out under pressure. This decreases the bisacromial diameter and facilitates delivery. But it is not easily carried out, and there is always a risk of injuring the various structures lying below it. As the number of maneuvers needed to relieve shoulder impaction increases, the incidence of neurological complication also increases proportionately. In a large multicenter study of 2018 cases of shoulder dystocia deliveries, all six cases of hypoxic-ischemic encephalopathy were associated with the use of more than five maneuvers, and the mean time between delivery of the head and the remainder of the body was 10.75 minutes (3–20 minutes) [30]. It is recommended to document simultaneously the significant facts, findings, various procedures carried out in management of dystocia, and its sequelae. Simulation drills and display of shoulder dystocia protocols in the delivery room are recommended to improve communication among the labor room team and effective use of maneuvers in order to decrease the incidence of BPI.

CONCLUSION

In spite of a number of well-known, documented predisposing factors of shoulder dystocia, accurate predictability of any one or a combination of these is not high so as to prevent this complication in vaginal delivery. Therefore, the attending obstetrician should be well versed in these risk factors in order to anticipate the occurrence in women at high risk. The labor room team members should have good communication, protocols for its management visibly displayed in the delivery room, and always be prepared to successfully manage if it happens. One should be alert to the possibility of shoulder dystocia in a woman if there is history of birth injury in an index delivery, estimated birth weight 4000 g or greater in subsequent pregnancy, gestational diabetes, high maternal BMI, and Latin American ethnicity. Simulation programs should be encouraged in both ongoing as well as continuing education for the obstetricians in order to have a good outcome if and when shoulder dystocia is encountered in vaginal delivery.

REFERENCES

1. Poujade O, Azria E, Ceccaldi PF et al. Prevention of shoulder dystocia: A randomized controlled trial to evaluate an obstetric maneuver. *Eur J Obstet Gynecol Reprod Biol*. 2018;227:52–9.
2. American College of Obstetricians and Gynecologists. Shoulder dystocia. Practice Bulletin No. 178. *Obstet Gynecol*. 2017;129: e123–33.
3. Royal College of Obstetricians and Gynaecologists (RCOG). *Shoulder Dystocia*. Green-top Guideline No. 42, 2nd ed. London, UK: RCOG; 2012, updated February 2017.
4. Gherman RB, Ouzounian JG, Incerpi MH, Goodwin TM. Symphyseal separation and transient femoral neuropathy associated with the McRoberts' maneuver. *Am J Obstet Gynecol*. 1998;178:609–10.
5. American College of Obstetricians and Gynecologists (ACOG). *Neonatal Brachial Plexus Palsy*. Washington, DC: ACOG; 2014.
6. Thompson KA, Satin AJ, Gherman RB. Spiral fracture of the radius: An unusual case of shoulder dystocia–associated morbidity. *Obstet Gynecol*. 2003;102:36–8.
7. Habek D. Transient recurrent laryngeal nerve paresis after shoulder dystocia. *Int J Gynecol Obstet*. 2015;130:87–8.
8. Gherman RB, Chauhan S, Ouzounian JG, Lerner H, Gonik B, Goodwin TM. Shoulder dystocia: The unpreventable obstetric emergency with empiric management guidelines. *Am J Obstet Gynecol*. 2006;195:657–72.
9. Menjou M, Mottram J, Petts C, Stoner R. Common intrapartum denominators of obstetric brachial plexus injury (OBPI). *NHSLA J*. 2003;2(Suppl):ii–viii.
10. Draycott T, Sanders C, Crofts J, Lloyd JA template for reviewing the strength of evidence for obstetric brachial plexus injury in clinical negligence claims. *Clin Risk*. 2008;14:96–100.
11. Nesbitt TS, Gilbert WM, Herrchen B. Shoulder dystocia and associated risk factors with macrosomic infants born in California. *Am J Obstet Gynecol*. 1998;179:476–80.
12. Gross TL, Sokol RJ, Williams T, Thompson K. Shoulder dystocia: A fetal-physician risk. *Am J Obstet Gynecol*. 1987;156:1408–18.

13. Baskett TF, Allen AC. Perinatal implications of shoulder dystocia. *Obstet Gynecol.* 1995;86:14–7.

14. Ouzounian JG, Korst LM, Miller DA, Lee RH. Brachial plexus palsy and shoulder dystocia: Obstetrical risk factors remain elusive. *Am J Perinatol.* 2013;30:303–7.

15. Ouzounian JG, Gherman RB. Shoulder dystocia: Are historic risk factors reliable predictors? *Am J Obstet Gynecol.* 2005;192:1933–5; discussion 1935–8.

16. Ouzounian JG, Gherman RB, Chauhan S, Battista LR, Lee RH. Recurrent shoulder dystocia: Analysis of incidence and risk factors. *Am J Perinatol.* 2012;29:515–8.

17. Dildy GA, Clark SL. Shoulder dystocia: Risk identification. *Clin Obstet Gynecol.* 2000;43:265.

18. McFarland MB, Trylovich CG, Langer O. Anthropometric differences in macrosomic infants of diabetic and nondiabetic mothers. *J Matern Fetal Med.* 1998;7:292.

19. Coustan DR, Lowe LP, Metzger BE et al. The Hyperglycemia and Adverse Pregnancy Outcome (HAPO) study: Paving the way for new diagnostic criteria for gestational diabetes mellitus. *Am J Obstet Gynecol.* 2010;202:654.e1.

20. Moore HM, Reed SD, Batra M, Schiff MA. Risk factors for recurrent shoulder dystocia, Washington state, 1987–2004. *Am J Obstet Gynecol.* 2008;198:e16.

21. Caughey AB, Sandberg PL, Zlatnik MG, Thiet MP, Parer JT, Laros RK Jr. Forceps compared with vacuum: Rates of neonatal and maternal morbidity. *Obstet Gynecol.* 2006;107:426–7.

22. Rouse DJ, Owen J, Goldenberg RL, Cliver SP. The effectiveness and costs of elective cesarean delivery for fetal macrosomia diagnosed by ultrasound. *JAMA.* 1996;276:1480.

23. Hehir MP, Mchugh AF, Maguire PJ, Mahony R. Extreme macrosomia—Obstetric outcomes and complications in birth weights >5000 g. *Aust N Z J Obstet Gynaecol.* 2015;55:42.

24. Boulvain M, Irion O, Dowswell T, Thornton JG. Induction of labour at or near term for suspected fetal macrosomia. *Cochrane Database Syst Rev.* 2016;(5):CD000938.

25. American College of Obstetricians and Gynecologists. Committee Opinion No. 765: Nonmedically Indicated Early-Term Deliveries and Associated Neonatal Morbidities (Joint with the Society for Maternal-Fetal Medicine). *Obstet Gynecol.* 2019;133:e156–63.

26. Caughey AB. Should pregnancies be induced for impending macrosomia? *Lancet.* 2015;385:2557–9.

27. Rodis JF. Shoulder dystocia: Risk factors and planning delivery of high-risk pregnancies. UpToDate Topic 4472 Version 27.0; 2019.

28. Sagi-Dain L, Sagi S. The role of episiotomy in prevention and management of shoulder dystocia: A systematic review. *Obstet Gynecol Surv.* 2015;70:354–62.

29. Gherman RB, Tramont J, Muffley P, Goodwin TM. Analysis of McRoberts' maneuver by x-ray pelvimetry. *Obstet Gynecol.* 2000;95:43–7.

30. Hoffman MK, Bailit JL, Branch DW et al. A comparison of obstetric maneuvers for the acute management of shoulder dystocia. *Obstet Gynecol.* 2011;117:1272–8.

31. Sandberg EC. The Zavanelli maneuver: 12 years of recorded experience. *Obstet Gynecol.* 1999:93:312–7.

32. O'Shaughnessy MJ. Hysterotomy facilitation of the vaginal delivery of the posterior arm in a case of severe shoulder dystocia. *Obstet Gynecol.* 1998;92:693–5.

33. Walsh JM, McAuliffe FM. Prediction and prevention of the macrosomic fetus. *Eur J Obstet Gynecol Reprod Biol.* 2012;162:125–30.

34. Hartling L, Dryden DM, Guthrie A et al. Benefits and harms of treating gestational diabetes mellitus: A systematic review and meta-analysis for the U.S. Preventive Services Task Force and the National Institutes of Health Office of Medical Applications of Research. *Ann Intern Med.* 2013;159:123.

35. Langer O, Rodriguez DA, Xenakis EM et al. Intensified versus conventional management of gestational diabetes. *Am J Obstet Gynecol.* 1994;170:1036.

36. McFarland M, Hod M, Piper JM, Xenakis EM, Langer O. Are labor abnormalities more common in shoulder dystocia? *Am J Obstet Gynecol.* 1995;173:1211–4.

37. Witkop CT, Neale D, Wilson LM et al. Active compared with expectant delivery management in women with gestational diabetes: A systematic review. *Obstet Gynecol.* 2009;113:206.

12

Management of pregnancy with one or more early neonatal deaths

RIMPI SINGLA

DEFINITION

Neonatal death is defined as the death of a live-born infant within the first 28 completed days of life, regardless of gestational age at birth [1]. This is further subdivided into early (deaths occurring between 0 and 7 days of birth) and late (deaths occurring after 7 days to 28 days of birth) neonatal deaths [2]. Neonatal death within the first 24 hours of life should be recorded in units of completed hours or minutes of life, while those occurring 24 hours of life or later should be recorded in units of completed days [3].

MAGNITUDE OF PROBLEM

The early neonatal period is the most critical period for survival. According to an estimate in 2013, the majority of neonatal deaths occur in the early neonatal period (36% within the first 24 hours and 37% between days 1 and 7 of life) [2]. Despite a decline in the neonatal mortality rate by more than 40% (from 31.9 to 18.4 deaths per 1000 live births) from 1990 to 2013 globally [4], this rate of decline is less than the decline in mortality in children of the age group of 1–59 months (56%) [2]. Hence, neonatal deaths are emerging as a major contributor to infant deaths. A UNICEF report in 2014 confirms the increase in the contribution of neonatal deaths toward the deaths reported in the under-5-year age group from 37.4% in 1990 to 41.6% in 2013 [2,4]. The focus should now shift to measures to reduce neonatal deaths. It is important to note that 97%–99% of all neonatal deaths globally occur in low- and middle-income countries (LMICs) [5]. Most stillbirths and neonatal deaths are preventable through improvements in antenatal and intrapartum care. This has been recognized in the third Sustainable Development Goal (SDG) that also states that the neonatal mortality rate should be reduced in all countries to at least 12 per 1000 live births [6].

CAUSES AND RISK FACTORS

The causes of stillbirth and early neonatal death are generally inseparable. Major ones accounting for most of the neonatal deaths include preterm birth (accounting for 30%), infections (27%), and birth asphyxia (23%) (Table 12.1) [7–10]. Others are congenital abnormalities (6%), neonatal tetanus (4%), diarrhea (3%), and other minor causes (7%) [9,10]. In India, the majority (78%) of neonatal deaths occur due to prematurity and low birth weight (LBW), infections, birth asphyxia, and birth trauma in descending order [11,12].

Table 12.1 Causes of early neonatal death

Causes	Immediate reason
Maternal	
Young maternal age	Prematurity and LBW
Maternal malnutrition	Prematurity and LBW
Maternal medical disorders (hypertension, diabetes mellitus, anemia, heart disease, etc.)	Placental insufficiency leading to prematurity, LBW, APH, birth defect
APLA syndrome	Placental insufficiency leading to prematurity, LBW
Antepartum hemorrhage	Hypovolemia, asphyxia
Placenta previa	
Abruptio placentae	
Maternal infections (malaria, syphilis)	Fetal infections, birth defects, prematurity
PPROM	Prematurity, neonatal infection
Preterm labor	Prematurity
Chorioamnionitis	Neonatal infection
Smoking and alcohol intake	Placental insufficiency, birth defects
Complications of labor and delivery	Birth asphyxia, birth trauma
Fetal and neonatal causes	
Prematurity	RDS (including HMD)
	IVH
	NEC
	Infections
Low birth weight	
Infections (pneumonia, meningitis, sepsis)	
Birth defects	
Disorders of metabolism	
Genetic disorders	
SIDS	

Abbreviations: APH, antepartum hemorrhage; APLA, antiphospholipid antibody syndrome; HMD, hyaline membrane disease; IVH, intraventricular hemorrhage; LBW, low birth weight; NEC, necrotizing enterocolitis; PPROM, preterm premature rupture of membranes; RDS, respiratory distress syndrome; SIDS, sudden infant death syndrome.

Immediate causes of death in premature neonates are respiratory distress syndrome, intraventricular hemorrhage, necrotizing enterocolitis, and infections (pneumonia, sepsis, and meningitis).

Birth asphyxia

Mortality due to birth asphyxia is largely related to a lack of antenatal and intrapartum care [8,13]. Hence, birth asphyxia (responsible for 35%–42%) and sepsis (28%) account for the majority of early neonatal deaths in LMIC countries like Bangladesh [14].

Birth defects

Common birth defects that lead to early neonatal death include heart anomalies (hypoplastic left heart syndrome, transposition of great vessels, critical pulmonary stenosis, interrupted aortic arch, myocardial infarction), genetic disorders, and neural tube defects. Other causes include disorders of metabolism (urea cycle defect, congenital lactic acidemia), hypovolemia (subgaleal hemorrhage, placenta previa, and placental abruption), and airway abnormalities (prolapsed epiglottis with laryngomalacia) [15].

Sudden infant death syndrome (SIDS)

Sometimes there is sudden and unexpected death of a newborn that is initially unexplained. When it remains unexplained despite thorough investigation, including review of clinical history, records, and autopsy, this is referred to as SIDS. Risk factors for SIDS include kangaroo care, mothers falling asleep while breastfeeding (due to fatigue and influences of analgesia), bed sharing, prone sleeping, and even being primigravid [16–18]. The majority of such collapses have been reported to occur between 11 p.m. and 6 a.m., and 77% of all events occur within the first 3 days of life. These can essentially be prevented by educating healthcare professionals and parents.

Maternal age

There is an inherent biological risk of early neonatal death associated with young maternal age (less than 20 years of age) that persists even after adjusting for socioeconomic and demographic factors [19,20]. Adolescent mothers are at a higher risk of having premature and LBW babies [21], due to nutritional insufficiencies, infections, and hypertension.

Maternal nutrition

Adequate maternal nutrition has been shown to be associated with a lower risk of neonatal death (adjusted odds ratio [OR] 0.4; 95% confidence interval [CI] 0.2, 0.8) [14].

Maternal obesity

Overweight and obese mothers have increased odds of experiencing perinatal death as compared to mothers with healthy body mass index (BMI). The odds are greatest for the most obese (BMI >35) [22,23].

A history of previous infant deaths, hospitalization during pregnancy, lack of ultrasound examination in the prenatal period, and transfer of the newborn to another unit have also been recognized as determining factors for neonatal death [24]. The World Health Organization's (WHO) Global Survey on Maternal and Perinatal Health conducted from 2004 to 2008 in 23 developing countries has shown that women whose first pregnancy ended in perinatal death (stillbirth or neonatal death) were more likely to experience similar outcome or give birth to a LBW infant or to have an infant requiring admission to the neonatal intensive care unit in their next pregnancy [25].

MANAGEMENT

Management of further pregnancy in a woman who has experienced previous early neonatal loss begins well before conception (Figure 12.1). Preconceptional counseling is important to identify the cause (if not known), determine the risk of recurrence, optimize maternal health, and make a plan for management in subsequent pregnancy.

In the preconceptional period, detailed history should be obtained, and records of the prenatal period of previous pregnancy should be reviewed, especially to check whether supervised or not, intake of folic acid, prenatal complications, and gestational age at delivery, that may be the actual cause or a contributory factor. Details of labor and delivery provide insight into intrapartum events that may be responsible for adverse perinatal outcome. The neonatologist's notes wherever available provide information on Apgar score, birth weight, approximate gestational age, need for resuscitation, intensive care unit care, feeding, and many other factors that help in future counseling. An autopsy gives additional information in at least one in three cases. Further information can be obtained from available genetic tests, x-rays, and tests on placenta and umbilical cord. Early neonatal deaths should always be classified using the *International Classification of Diseases, Tenth Revision–Perinatal Mortality* (ICD-PM) classification. *ICD-PM* guides health-care providers in correctly documenting pertinent information, as it clarifies which conditions should be considered as underlying causes of death and thus helps in identifying the attributable cause. Correct classification based on underlying neonatal and maternal causes of death helps in finding the risk of recurrence.

Specific interventions in preconceptional time

The preconceptional period is the ideal time to optimize maternal illnesses that could affect

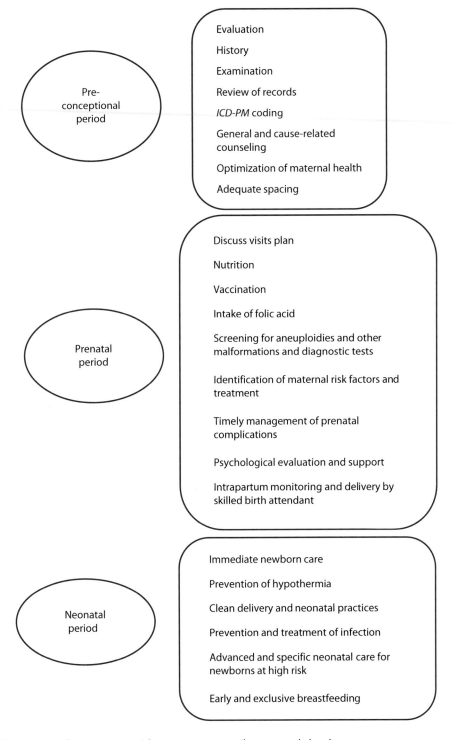

Figure 12.1 Approach to women with one or more early neonatal deaths.

pregnancy outcome, as treatment is not surrounded by the fear of teratogenicity. For example, hypertension and diabetes, established risk factors for adverse perinatal outcome, should be brought under control. Diet and exercise plans should be discussed and emphasized in order to optimize maternal weight. A consultation with a dietician is helpful. Known autoimmune disorders should be treated such that conception occurs in a remission phase. Due care should be given to contraception if a patient is having disease flare. Such a woman should be investigated for secondary antiphospholipid antibody (APLA) syndrome and a treatment plan for pregnancy formulated accordingly.

Periconceptual folic acid supplementation

Intake of folic acid prior to conception through 3 months after conception is associated with a reduction in the risk of neural tube defects (NTDs). For this, all women planning pregnancy should consume 400 mcg of folic acid per day [26].

Genetic counseling

Women with previous neonatal loss attributable to genetic disorders should be counseled by a geneticist. It is ideal to know a diagnosis for appropriate genetic counseling, but this is not available in most cases. This also helps in knowing the risk of recurrence. Women with known familial disorders or known genetic disorder in a previous child should be offered prenatal or preimplantation genetic diagnosis, as applicable and locally available.

Interconceptual interval

Birth spacing should be carefully planned as both too short (less than 18 months) and too long (greater than 60 months) interpregnancy intervals are associated with adverse perinatal outcomes, especially small for gestational age (SGA) babies [27]. A birth interval of less than 18 months has been shown to be associated with increased odds of SGA, preterm, and mortality as compared to that of 36 to less than 60 months. A birth interval at the other end of the spectrum (more than 60 months) has also increased risk for an SGA baby [27,28].

Interventions during pregnancy

High neonatal mortality in developing countries despite receiving intensive care unit care as compared to developed countries highlights the importance of care in the prenatal period [29,30] (Table 12.2). Adequate prenatal care identifies and resolves maternal and fetal complications and, hence, has a key role in preventing LBW and prematurity [8,30,31]. This further translates into a reduction in neonatal mortality [31].

Number of prenatal visits

Women having more prenatal visits have lower neonatal morbidity and mortality. Perinatal mortality has been shown to increase with a reduction in the number of prenatal visits, especially in LMICs [32]. The quality of care provided during prenatal visits is important. The focus of prenatal care visits should be on delivering effective, appropriate, and timely screening and diagnostic, preventive, and therapeutic interventions [26].

Iron supplementation during pregnancy for maternal anemia

Iron deficiency anemia in the mother increases the risk of preterm birth and LBW and, hence, increases the risk of neonatal death [33]. Iron supplements are known to reduce the risk of having LBW newborns (below 2500 g) [34].

Calcium supplementation

Women with high dietary calcium intake have a lower prevalence of preeclampsia [35]. Calcium supplementation has been shown to reduce the risk of preeclampsia (relative risk 0.45; 95% CI: 0.31, 0.65) [36].

Vaccination in pregnancy

Tetanus toxoid causes a reduction in mortality related to neonatal tetanus by 94% [37,38]. Currently, tetanus and influenza vaccines are widely recommended, and several countries also recommend vaccination against pertussis. Other vaccines being developed for use in pregnancy are against group B streptococcus, respiratory syncytial virus, and cytomegalovirus.

Table 12.2 Cause-specific management in subsequent pregnancy

	Causes	Preventive measures in next pregnancy
Prematurity and low birth weight	Induced preterm delivery Hypertension Fetal growth restriction Maternal medical disorders (heart disease, asthma, connective tissue disorders)	Control of disease (optimization of maternal condition) in preconceptional period Folic acid intake Low-dose aspirin LMWH in prophylactic dose for APLA syndrome Calcium supplementation Iron supplementation Continued medical management of disease Antenatal steroids if preterm delivery anticipated
	Spontaneous preterm labor PPROM	Progesterone support (natural micronized progesterone) Screening for GBS, STIs, and treatment Antenatal steroids if preterm delivery anticipated
Infections	Chorioamnionitis Maternal sepsis (all causes) Tropical fever TORCH infections	Generally nonrecurrent Malaria prophylaxis and preventive measures in endemic zones Vaccination Testing for syphilis and treatment Treatment of risk factors such as diabetes, anemia
	Neonatal sepsis Pneumonia Meningitis Tetanus	Infection prevention measures universally Clean delivery and neonatal practices Hand hygiene Chlorhexidine rubs Cord care Maternal vaccination
Birth asphyxia	Lack of intrapartum monitoring/ facilities to expedite delivery Lack of skilled birth attendant Lack of immediate newborn care Birth trauma	Facility-based measures Better antenatal care Labor and delivery in center equipped with facilities and trained staff for intrapartum surveillance, instrumental delivery and caesarean section, and newborn care and resuscitation Screening and treatment of diabetes
Birth defects	Malformations Genetic disorders	Periconceptional folic acid Diagnosis of previous child and counseling according to risk of recurrence Preimplantation genetic diagnosis/prenatal diagnosis First-trimester ultrasound for aneuploidy screening Ultrasound in second trimester for malformations including echocardiography Early saturation screening of the newborn

Abbreviations: APLA, antiphospholipid antibody syndrome; GBS, Group B Streptococcus; LMWH, low molecular weight heparin; PPROM, preterm premature rupture of membranes; STI, sexually transmitted infection; TORCH, toxoplasmosis, other (syphilis), rubella, cytomegalovirus, herpes simplex virus.

Prevention of infectious diseases

This is particularly important in tropical countries. In malaria endemic zones, the WHO has suggested use of insecticide-treated nets and antimalarial drugs (for prophylactic and therapeutic use) in pregnancy [39]. Prophylaxis with sulfadoxine-pyrimethamine reduces prenatal parasitemia and, hence, reduces LBW. Maternal syphilis is known to result in fetal malformations and adverse perinatal outcomes, and its treatment is associated with reduction in the same and neonatal mortality [40].

Management of preterm premature rupture of membranes

Women with a history of neonatal death due to preterm birth have been shown to benefit by progesterone support. Premature rupture of membranes complicates 5%–10% of all pregnancies. When expectant management is preferred, antibiotics should be administered in order to reduce the chances of chorioamnionitis [41], preterm birth, respiratory distress syndrome (RDS), and early-onset postnatal infection including pneumonia and reduced neonatal mortality [42]. Prenatal corticosteroids bring about a significant reduction in the incidence of RDS and cerebroventricular hemorrhage [43] among preterm infants. Randomized controlled trials in middle-income countries suggest reductions in mortality and morbidity by 53% and 37%, respectively [44].

Antiplatelet agents

Low-dose aspirin has been shown to prevent or delay the onset of preeclampsia. This transforms into reduction in uteroplacental insufficiency and fetal growth retardation, and preterm birth associated with hypertensive disorders. Aspirin causes significant reduction in all types of deaths (fetal, neonatal, infant). Women who have gestational hypertension benefit even more due to reduction in preeclampsia [45]. In the event of early neonatal death owing to prematurity due to severe preeclampsia or placental insufficiency, women should be tested for APLA syndrome. They should be diagnosed with APLA syndrome if lupus anticoagulant is present or if anticardiolipin antibodies (immunoglobulin G [IgG] or IgM) are present in a titer of greater than 20 binding units. Women with APLA syndrome should receive low molecular weight heparin in a prophylactic dose and low-dose aspirin during

pregnancy. This reduces the risks of preeclampsia, placental insufficiency, and preterm birth. These women should also be considered for antepartum testing after 32 weeks (or earlier if indicated) [46].

Birth defects

Screening and diagnostic tests for aneuploidies and fetal anomaly scans during pregnancy and a comprehensive clinical examination of the newborn can prevent the majority of neonatal deaths due to cardiac disease and/or persistent pulmonary hypertension. Saturation screening in newborns detects congenital heart disease, pulmonary disease, and maladaptation associated with transition from fetal to neonatal circulation and ensures timely management [47].

Smoking cessation

Smoking cessation strategies including counseling, cognitive behavioral therapy, nicotine replacement therapy, and bupropion and social support are associated with a reduction in LBW and preterm birth [48].

Psychological aspects

Subsequent pregnancies following early neonatal death are surrounded by uncertainties, insecurities, maternal anxiety, and emotional instability. Emotional vulnerability often extends beyond the postpartum period resulting in disrupted attachment, potentially leading to parenting and social difficulties in the long term [49,50]. Some women who conceive within 5–6 months of perinatal loss exhibit inappropriate grief responses. Identifying the cause of death and counseling accordingly decrease the intensity of grief and feeling of self-blame, but insecurities over outcome in subsequent pregnancy remain. This demands additional emotional and psychological support from healthcare providers [51].

Feasible preventive care in low-resource settings

Apart from adequate prenatal care, neonatal mortality can be further reduced by improvements in intrapartum care (availability of skilled birth attendant, emergency obstetric care, immediate and effective newborn care, and functional referral system), clean delivery and neonatal care practices (clean cord cutting, hand hygiene, using chlorhexidine), and postnatal continued family-community care. In low-resource settings, services of general health workers and traditional birth attendants can be utilized in effectively delivering intrapartum care and management of sepsis [52–54]. Home-based management of LBW and preterm neonates with treatment of infections, promotion of early and exclusive breastfeeding, and prevention of hypothermia, including kangaroo mother care, are effective in improving neonatal survival [54–56].

CONCLUSION

With a decline in deaths between 1 month and 5 years, neonatal deaths are emerging as an important cause of under-5-year mortality. Early neonatal deaths are largely preventable, as most important causes are related to prenatal and intrapartum care. Most important causes include prematurity, birth asphyxia, and infections. The optimization of maternal health and control of preexisting diseases prior to conception, comprehensive prenatal care with timely referral and management of high-risk pregnancies, intrapartum care including vigilant fetal monitoring, and immediate newborn resuscitation and prevention of infections are key to the reduction of early neonatal losses and their recurrence.

REFERENCES

1. World Health Organization (WHO). *Neonatal and Perinatal Mortality: Country, Regional and Global Estimates*. Geneva, Switzerland: WHO; 2006. https://apps.who.int/iris/handle/10665/43444
2. UNICEF, WHO, World Bank, UN-DESA Population Division. *Levels and trends in child mortality*. Report. New York, NY; 2014.
3. International Statistical Classification of Diseases and Related Health Problems-10th Revision (ICD-10); World Health Organization. 2011;2:195. (International Classification of Diseases [ICD]. Instruction Manual. 6 Classifications.)
4. GBD 2013 Mortality and Causes of Death Collaborators. Global, regional, and national age-sex specific all-cause and cause-specific mortality for 240 causes of death, 1990–2013: A systematic analysis for the Global Burden of Disease Study 2013. *Lancet*. 2015;385(9963):117–71.
5. Liu L, Johnson HL, Cousens S et al. Child Health Epidemiology Reference Group of WHO and UNICEF. Global, regional, and national causes of child mortality: An updated systematic analysis for 2010 with time trends since 2000. *Lancet*. 2012;379:2151–61.
6. Taylor S, Williams B, Magnus D, Goenka A, Modi N. From MDG to SDG: Good news for global child health? *The Lancet*. 2015;386:1213–4.
7. Rajaratnam JK, Marcus JR, Flaxman AD et al. Neonatal, postneonatal, childhood, and under 5 mortality for 187 countries, 1970–2010: A systematic analysis of progress towards Millennium Development Goal 4. *Lancet*. 2010;375:1988–2008.
8. Schoeps D, Furquim de Almeida M, Alencar GP et al. Risk factors for early neonatal mortality. *Rev Saude Publica*. 2007;41:1013–22.
9. World Health Organization (WHO). *The World Health Report: 2005: Make Every Mother and Child Count*. Geneva, Switzerland: WHO; 2005: 219.
10. Bryce J, Boschi-Pinto C, Shibuya K, Black RE, WHO Child Health Epidemiology Reference Group. WHO estimates of the causes of death in children. *Lancet*. 2005;365:1147–52.
11. Million Death Study Collaborators, Bassani DG, Kumar R et al. Causes of neonatal and child mortality in India: A nationally representative mortality survey. *Lancet*. 2010;376(9755):1853–60.
12. Fottrell E, Osrin D, Alcock G et al. Cause-specific neonatal mortality: Analysis of 3772 neonatal deaths in Nepal, Bangladesh, Malawi and India. *Arch Dis Child Fetal Neonatal Ed*. 2015;100:F439–47.
13. Lansky S, França E, Kawachi I. Social inequalities in perinatal mortality in Belo Horizonte, Brazil: The role of hospital care. *Am J Public Health*. 2007;97:867–73.
14. Owais A, Faruque ASG, Das SK et al. Maternal and antenatal risk factors for stillbirths and neonatal mortality in rural Bangladesh: A case-control study. *PLOS ONE*. 2013;8(11):e80164.
15. Lutz TL, Elliott EJ, Jeffery HE. Sudden unexplained early neonatal death or collapse: A national surveillance study. *Pediatr Res*. 2016;80(4): 493–8.

16. Thach BT. Deaths and near deaths of healthy newborn infants while bed sharing on maternity wards. *J Perinatol.* 2014;34:275–9.

17. Herlenius E, Kuhn P. Sudden unexpected postnatal collapse of newborn infants: A review of cases, definitions, risks, and preventive measures. *Transl Stroke Res.* 2013;4:236–47.

18. Dageville C, Pignol J, De Smet S. Very early neonatal apparent life-threatening events and sudden unexpected deaths: Incidence and risk factors. *Acta Paediatr.* 2008;97:866–9.

19. Neal S, Channon AA, Chintsanya J. The impact of young maternal age at birth on neonatal mortality: Evidence from 45 low and middle income countries. *PLOS ONE.* 2018;13(5):e0195731.

20. Sharma V, Katz J, Mullany LC et al. Young maternal age and the risk of neonatal mortality in rural Nepal. *Arch Pediatr Adolesc Med.* 2008;162(9):828–35.

21. Chen X-K, Wen SW, Fleming N, Yang Q, Walker MC. Increased risks of neonatal and postneonatal mortality associated with teenage pregnancy had different explanations. *J Clin Epidemiol.* 2008;61(7):688–94.

22. Meehan S, Beck CR, Mair-Jenkins J, Leonardi-Bee J, Puleston R. Maternal obesity and infant mortality: A meta-analysis. *Pediatrics.* 2014;133;863.

23. Tennant PW, Rankin J, Bell R. Maternal body mass index and the risk of fetal and infant death: A cohort study from the North of England. *Hum Reprod.* 2011;26(6):1501–11.

24. Kassar SB, Melo AM, Coutinho SB, Lima MC, Lira PI. Determinants of neonatal death with emphasis on health care during pregnancy, childbirth and reproductive history. *J Pediatr.* 2013;89:269–77.

25. Ouyang F, Zhang J, Betrán AP et al. Recurrence of adverse perinatal outcomes in developing countries. *Bull World Health Organ.* 2013;91:357–67.

26. Lassi ZS, Mansoor T, Salam RA et al. Pregnancy interventions: Essential prepregnancy and pregnancy interventions for improved maternal, newborn and child health. *Reprod Health.* 2014;11(Suppl 1):S2.

27. Conde-Agudelo A, Rosas-Bermudez A, Kafury-Goeta AC. Birth spacing and risk of adverse perinatal outcomes. *JAMA.* 2006;295(15):1809–23.

28. Kozuki N, Lee ACC, Silveira MF et al. The associations of birth intervals with small-for-gestational-age, preterm, and neonatal and infant mortality: A meta-analysis. *BMC Public Health.* 2013;13(Suppl 3):S3.

29. Castro EC, Leite AJ. Hospital mortality rates of infants with birth weight less than or equal to 1,500 g in the northeast of Brazil. *J Pediatr.* 2007;83:27–32.

30. Almeida MF, Guinsburg R, Martinez FE et al. Perinatal factors associated with early deaths of preterm infants born in Brazilian network on neonatal research centers. *J Pediatr.* 2008;84:300–7.

31. Darmstadt GL, Bhutta ZA, Cousens S et al. Evidence-based, cost-effective interventions: How many newborn babies can we save? *Lancet.* 2005;365:977–88.

32. Dowswell T, Carroli G, Duley L et al. Alternative versus standard packages of antenatal care for low-risk pregnancy. *Cochrane Database Syst Rev.* 2010;10(10):CD000934.

33. Scholl TO, Hediger ML, Fischer RL, Shearer JW. Anemia vs iron deficiency: Increased risk of preterm delivery in a prospective study. *Am J Clin Nutr.* 1992;55(5):985–8.

34. Pena-Rosas J, De-Regil L, Dowswell T, Viteri F. Daily oral iron supplementation during pregnancy. *Cochrane Database Syst Rev.* 2012;12(12):CD004736.

35. Belizán JM, Villar J, Bergel E, González L, Campodónico L. Calcium supplementation to prevent hypertensive disorders of pregnancy. *NEJM.* 1991;325:1399–405.

36. Imdad A, Jabeen A, Bhutta ZA. Role of calcium supplementation during pregnancy in reducing risk of developing gestational hypertensive disorders: A meta-analysis of studies from developing countries. *BMC Public Health.* 2011;11(Suppl 3):S18.

37. Blencowe H, Lawn J, Vandelaer J, Roper M, Cousens S. Tetanus toxoid immunization to reduce mortality from neonatal tetanus. *Int J Epidemiol.* 2010;39(Suppl 1):i102–9.

38. Demicheli V, Barale A, Rivetti A. Vaccines for women to prevent neonatal tetanus. *Cochrane Database Syst Rev.* 2013;5(5):CD002959.

39. Gamble C, Ekwaru PJ, Garner P, ter Kuile FO. Insecticide-treated nets for the prevention of malaria in pregnancy: A systematic review

of randomised controlled trials. *PLOS Med* 2007;4(3):e107.

40. Blencowe H, Cousens S, Kamb M, Berman S, Lawn JE. Lives saved tool supplement detection and treatment of syphilis in pregnancy to reduce syphilis related stillbirths and neonatal mortality. *BMC Public Health.* 2011;11(Suppl 3):S9.

41. Kenyon S, Boulvain M, Neilson JP. Antibiotics for preterm rupture of membranes. *Cochrane Database Syst Rev.* 2010;8(8):CD001058.

42. Cousens S, Blencowe H, Gravett M, Lawn JE. Antibiotics for pre-term prelabour rupture of membranes: Prevention of neonatal deaths due to complications of pre-term birth and infection. *Int J Epidemiol.* 2010;39(Suppl 1):i134–43.

43. Roberts D, Dalziel S. Antenatal corticosteroids for accelerating fetal lung maturation for women at risk of preterm birth. *Cochrane Database Syst Rev.* 2006;3(3):CD004454.

44. Mwansa-Kambafwile J, Cousens S, Hansen T, Lawn JE. Antenatal steroids in preterm labour for the prevention of neonatal deaths due to complications of preterm birth. *Int J Epidemiol.* 2010;39(Suppl 1):i122–33.

45. Duley L, Henderson-Smart DJ, Meher S, King JF. Antiplatelet agents for preventing pre-eclampsia and its complications. *Cochrane Database Syst Rev.* 2007;4(4):CD004659.

46. Committee on Practice Bulletins—Obstetrics, American College of Obstetricians and Gynecologists. Practice bulletin no. 132: Antiphospholipid syndrome. *Obstet Gynecol.* 2012;120(6):1514–21.

47. Meberg A, Brügmann-Pieper S, Due R Jr et al. First day of life pulse oximetry screening to detect congenital heart defects. *J Pediatr.* 2008;152:761–5.

48. Lumley J, Chamberlain C, Dowswell T, Oliver S, Oakley L, Watson L. Interventions for promoting smoking cessation during pregnancy. *Cochrane Database Syst Rev.* 2009;3(3):CD001055.

49. Hughes PM, Turton P, Evans CD. Stillbirth as risk factor for depression and anxiety in the subsequent pregnancy: Cohort study. *BMJ.* 1999;318(7200):1721–4.

50. Warland J, O'Leary J, McCutcheon H, Williamson V. Parenting paradox: Parenting after infant loss. *Midwifery.* 2011;27(5):e163–69.

51. Mills TA, Ricklesford C, Cooke A, Heazell AE, Whitworth M, Lavender T. Parents' experiences and expectations of care in pregnancy after stillbirth or neonatal death: A metasynthesis. *BJOG.* 2014;121(8):943–50.

52. Wall SN, Lee AC, Niermeyer S et al. Neonatal resuscitation in low-resource settings: What, who, and how to overcome challenges to scale up? *Int J Gynaecol Obstet.* 2009;107(Suppl 1):S47–62. S63–4.

53. Bang AT, Bang RA, Baitule SB, Reddy MH, Deshmukh MD. Effect of home-based neonatal care and management of sepsis on neonatal mortality: Field trial in rural India. *Lancet.* 1999;354:1955–61.

54. Bhutta ZA, Darmstadt GL, Hasan BS, Haws RA. Community-based interventions for improving perinatal and neonatal health outcomes in developing countries: A review of the evidence. *Pediatrics.* 2005;115(2 Suppl):519–617.

55. McClure EM, Goldenberg RL, Brandes N, CHX Working Group et al. The use of chlorhexidine to reduce maternal and neonatal mortality and morbidity in low-resource settings. *Int J Gynaecol Obstet.* 2007;97:89–94.

56. World Health Organization. Collaborative Study Team. Effect of breastfeeding on infant and child mortality due to infectious diseases in less developed countries: A pooled analysis. WHO Collaborative Study Team on the Role of Breastfeeding on the Prevention of Infant Mortality. *Lancet.* 2000;355:451–5.

13

Management of pregnancy with a history of late neonatal/infant death

DARSHAN HOSAPATNA BASAVARAJAPPA

INTRODUCTION

Every pregnant woman wishes for a healthy newborn and to cherish the happiness for her lifetime, but if a newborn succumbs to a disease or a disorder, great agony is experienced. The psychological and financial impact on the woman and her family is indescribable. With expectations for a healthy baby and continuing apprehension during her pregnancy, detailed evaluation and holistic care are essential for a favorable maternal and neonatal outcome.

The neonatal period includes the time period between birth and 28 days of life. It has been further subdivided into early neonatal, comprising the first 6 days; late neonatal, from 7 to 28 days; and infancy, for the first year of life [1]. This division not only serves a statistical purpose but also helps in analyzing different causes and cause-specific interventions to combat future adversities. In general, early neonatal mortalities are the consequences of pregnancy and labor complications. They reflect the prenatal care and labor facilities and immediate postpartum and neonatal care that the women received. Late neonatal deaths are supposed to be the result of child-specific entities.

The World Health Organization (WHO) estimates that around 2.5 million children died in the first 28 days of life in the year 2017. A child's risk of dying is highest in the first 28 days of life, during the neonatal period. In 2017, 47% of all under-5-year child deaths were neonatal deaths, which was 40% in 1990 [2]. Children who die in the neonatal period suffer from conditions and diseases associated with a lack of prenatal care or in adequate labor facilities and postpartum treatment. In countries with high under-5-year mortality indices, perinatal mortality and infant mortality rates are also rising. Hence, knowledge of common causes of neonatal and infant deaths is useful in analyzing specific approaches to such mishaps.

Table 13.1 lists a few of the important causes of early and late neonatal mortalities. There are different proportions of contribution in both periods. Hence, there arises the need to identify clear causes of mortality and significant measures to avoid those in future pregnancies.

Table 13.1 Global cause-specific numbers of neonatal deaths, proportions and risks in 2013

Cause	Early neonatal period		Late neonatal period	
	Number of deaths in thousands	Proportion (%)	Number of deaths in thousands	Proportion (%)
Preterm birth	834.8	40.8	152.1	21.2
Intrapartum complications	552.7	27	92.1	12.9
Congenital disorders	217	10.6	72.8	10.2
Sepsis	163.7	8	266.7	37.2
Pneumonia	98.9	4.8	37.6	5.2
Diarrhea	6.7	0.3	10	1.4
Tetanus	21.1	1	27.1	3.8
Others	149.9	7.3	57.9	8.1

Source: Oza S et al. Bull World Health Organ. 2015;93(1):19–28.

APPROACH TO WOMEN WITH PREVIOUS LATE NEONATAL DEATH

Many of the pregnant women who visit the prenatal clinic in their early pregnancy with a history of previous neonatal deaths usually carry details and hospital records with information regarding the neonatal disease. These details must be utilized completely in addressing the issue.

The following questions are helpful in the obstetric history for discovering the cause:

1. Was the problem identified in previous pregnancy or after the delivery of the child?
2. Were there any intrapartum difficulties, and what was the mode of delivery?
3. What was the birth weight of the previous child?
4. Were the Apgar scores and cries of the baby optimal?
5. What was the duration of the nursery or neonatal intensive care unit stay?
6. What was the duration between onset of disease and critical illness or death?
7. Were any medical or surgical interventions done?
8. Are special investigations like karyotype or genetic analysis available?

With answers to the majority of questions, a reasonable approach can be devised and appropriate steps taken. Most of the neonatal diseases are non-recurrent and mostly influenced by environmental and social causes (Figure 13.1). One particular cause may not be possibly isolated in many situations. In such instances, a thorough genetic evaluation by a geneticist will contribute to the management. Ideal prenatal and intrapartum care will suffice for a favorable maternal and neonatal outcome.

The three important causes of recurrent neonatal deaths worthy of discussion are

1. *Congenital malformations*: Not lethal enough to cause death immediately but morbidly serious

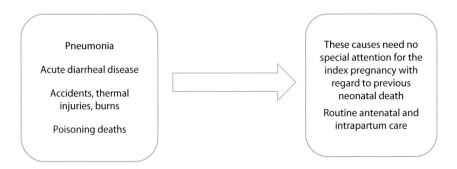

Figure 13.1 Major nonrecurrent neonatal illnesses and the approach in subsequent pregnancies.

2. *Inborn errors of metabolism*: Most important recurrent cause; usually unidentified if not picked up early by subtle signs
3. *Late-onset neonatal sepsis*: A cause usually secondary to prematurity complications and hospital-acquired infections

CONGENITAL MALFORMATIONS

Congenital malformations can be lethal enough that they are incompatible with life or may be insignificant. Lethal malformations lead to intra-uterine deaths or early neonatal mortalities when not treated or when corrected ineffectively. But, many times parents agree to the treatment and correction of deformities and malformations, and this sometimes leads to failed attempts, and the neonate succumbs to further complications.

Chromosomal aneuploidies and syndromic manifestations also add up to growth restriction, prematurity, further sepsis, and neurologic mor-bidities. Hence, detailed knowledge of the affected malformations of the previous child can help in assigning the cause and delineating the inheri-tance patterns, and possibly lead to avoidance of the recurrence or, if identified, to early termination of pregnancies medically.

Although around 50% of all congenital anoma-lies are sporadic, there are some known genetic, environmental, and other causes.

Genetic factors

Genetic factors are the most important cause for certain congenital anomalies. There can be inheri-tance by Mendelian genetics or mutations that can result in the manifestation. Consanguinity contributes significantly to genetic manifestations and their inheritance, leading to an increased risk of neonatal mortality, intellectual disability, and physical handicaps. Some families and geographic ethnicities have predispositions to disorders, like Ashkenazi Jews and the royal family of England with hemophilia.

Socioeconomic and demographic factors

Malnutrition disorders and infections are not the only burdens imposed on low socioeco-nomic nations, but around 94% of congenital anomalies are witnessed in this group of nations. Lack of health education and awareness among reproductive-age women restricts them from basic commodities like nutritious food, micronutrients, folic acid supplements, iodinated salt, and early identification of problems by ultrasonography examinations. Neural tube defects and congeni-tal hypothyroidism are grave examples of poor maternal nutrition. To add to these adversities, unsafe drinking water and polluted food carrying industrial waste and heavy metals are potential teratogens for the growing fetus. Toxoplasmosis, congenital rubella syndrome, and fetal alcohol syndrome are the other such anomalies that can be prevented by proper health education and a global public health perspective.

Environmental factors

Pesticides and other chemical fertilizers, terato-genic drugs, alcohol, and radiation exposure dur-ing pregnancy may increase the risk of congenital anomalies.

Infections

Vertical transmission and perinatal transmission of infections is another important source of birth defects in newborns. Proper infection screening of expectant mothers and their treatment could potentially avoid these defects. Congenital syphi-lis, rubella syndrome, toxoplasmosis, and cyto-megalovirus infections are a few infections that can be screened for in expectant mothers.

A recent survey on trends and characteristics of fetal and neonatal mortality due to congeni-tal anomalies was conducted in Colombia from 1999 to 2008 and published in 2018 [4]. Various congenital malformations accounted for a pro-portion of neonatal mortalities as summarized in Table 13.2.

INBORN ERRORS OF METABOLISM

Inborn errors of metabolism (IEMs) form a large class of genetic disorders that occur as a result of gene defects. The majority are due to defects of single genes coding for enzymes. The identification of an IEM as a disorder in neonates was described in the early twentieth century. First, the disease known as alkaptonuria was discovered by Archibald Garrod,

Table 13.2 Common congenital malformations and proportion of neonatal mortality

Common congenital malformations	System-specific disorders	Proportion of neonatal mortality (%)
Congenital heart defects	Usually unspecific and complex congenital defects, hypoplastic left heart, ventricular septal defect, aortic coarctation	45
Central nervous system	Anencephaly, spina bifida and encephalocele, hydrocephalus and brain hypoplasia	14.1
Chromosomal	Edwards and Patau syndrome	2.2
Musculoskeletal system	Lethal skeletal dysplasia and achondroplasia	7.1
Digestive system	Tracheoesophageal fistulas, duodenal and jejunal atresia	6.7
Respiratory system	Airway obstruction syndromes and pulmonary hypoplasias	4.6
Urinary system	Bladder extrophy, renal agenesis, multicystic dysplastic kidneys, polycystic kidneys, bladder outlet obstruction	3.3
Orofacial clefts		0.2
Visual, auditory		0.01
Genital organs		0.01
Other	Hemoglobinopathies, single-gene disorders	16.7

in 1908 [5], followed by research in 1917 regarding the advice of less intake of milk by galactosemic infants, but the treatment of various disorders of IEMs changed in the 1950s with phenylketonuria.

IEMs are the most important cause of neonatal illness, and many of these disorders are treatable if diagnosed in the early stages. The failure to recognize subtle signs of inborn errors could lead to fatal neonatal disease and nonsalvage. Usually parents think excessive crying, fatigability, food intolerance, and sleeplessness as being normal neonatal behavior, but these could be early signs of metabolic disorders.

In poorly informed patients and underdeveloped countries, successive neonatal deaths are reported due to failure of recognition and treatment, caused secondary to lack of newborn screening facilities and specific treatment and superimposed sepsis.

Common signs of metabolic disorders that should trigger evaluation are as follows:

1. Poor suckling, excessive crying, and convulsions
2. Hypoglycemia, metabolic acidosis, jaundice, diarrhea, and vomiting
3. Hepatomegaly or splenomegaly, cataract, and apnea [6]

Common IEM disorders include

1. Amino acid disorders
2. Fatty acid oxidation disorders
3. Storage disorders, including both carbohydrate and lysosomal disorders
4. Organic acid disorders

LATE-ONSET NEONATAL SEPSIS

The incidence of late-onset neonatal sepsis (LONS) is inversely related to the degree of fetal maturity and varies geographically from 0.61% to 14.2% among hospitalized newborns [7].

Due to the difficulties in making a prompt diagnosis of LONS and the high risk of mortality and long-term neurodevelopmental sequelae associated with LONS, empirical antibiotic treatment is initiated on suspicion of LONS.

In contrast to early-onset neonatal sepsis, late-onset neonatal sepsis is not typically related to pregnancy and labor complications. Prematurity and respiratory diseases of newborns mandating invasive ventilation and unhygienic newborn handling are the most important factors responsible for LONS.

Risk factors for late-onset neonatal sepsis

Prematurity either directly by the process of acquiring maternal tract infections or indirectly as a consequence of prolonged hospitalization, interventions, intravenous catheters, and parenteral nutrition contributes to neonatal sepsis [8]. The fatality rate is two to four times higher in infants with low birth weight than in full-term infants. The overall mortality rate of early-onset sepsis is 3%–40% and of late-onset sepsis is 2%–20%.

Other causes

Other rare causes of neonatal mortality include neonatal tetanus, neonatal jaundice, hemorrhagic disease of the newborn, and term baby dying due to *in utero* growth restriction and its consequences. These need individualization of every case and appropriate management.

MANAGEMENT OF PREGNANCY WITH A HISTORY OF LATE NEONATAL DEATH

These patients have to be offered preconceptional counseling and preferably be supervised in high-risk pregnancy units with a team composed of an experienced obstetrician, a pediatrician, and a geneticist. A high degree of vigilance has to be ensured at all levels of pregnancy, during labor, and in the postpartum period. A thorough preconceptional approach and appropriate measures needs to be discussed in women with previous late neonatal death (Figure 13.2).

At first visit in early pregnancy

There is a preferred order for routine prenatal investigations, such as blood grouping and RhD typing and indirect Coombs test (ICT) titers if already Rh isoimmunized or in a previous hydrops fetalis or hemolytic jaundice–related death. Maternal thyroid function tests and antithyroid peroxidase are important assays in neonates with congenital hypothyroidism and mental retardation.

First-trimester glucose tolerance test or HbA1c levels in pregestational diabetics would guide further glycemic management and avoidance of hyperglycemia-induced malformations such as neural tube defects and conotruncal heart abnormalities.

Infection screening of rubella IgM and IgG and treponema screening tests are also part of the management. Institute routine supplementation of folic acid 5 mg in previous neural tube affected neonates

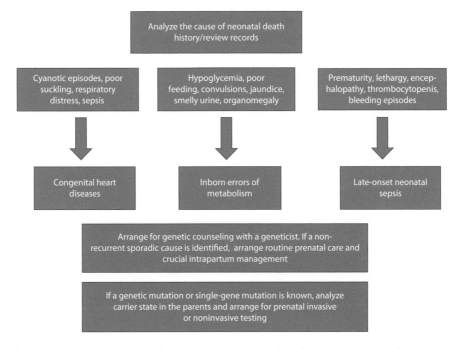

Figure 13.2 Preconceptional approach to women with previous late neonatal death.

and avoid any other teratogenic drugs or radiation exposure.

Pyrexia in the organogenesis period is also a contributory factor for malformations, and appropriate measures should be taken if there is maternal fever in early gestation.

Routine use of progestogens and aspirin in pregnancies with previous late neonatal death per se is not advised unless otherwise indicated.

At 8–10 weeks

Continue routine antepartum care.

Noninvasive prenatal testing for Down syndrome can be planned at this gestation if previous Down syndrome or if affected by any other aneuploidy.

At 11–13 weeks

Aneuploidy screening can be conducted. Combined screening of first-trimester biochemical screening (dual marker) and nuchal translucency with maternal age fairly estimates aneuploidy of trisomy 13, 18, and 21.

First-trimester sonography would scan for anencephaly, encephalocele, spina bifida, and major anomalies. Recurrent neural tube defects are sometimes associated with single-gene polymorphisms and can be picked up early.

Invasive prenatal testing in the form of chorionic villus sampling is scheduled at this gestation for detection of inheritable gene mutations and certain structural hemoglobinopathies.

At 16–20 weeks

This is the time for a detailed malformation scan by an experienced sonologist, which could elucidate all the anomalies, and a fetal echocardiography would effectively pick up structural heart defects.

Second-trimester aneuploidy screening can be done if first-trimester combined screening was missed or an integrated screening methodology is implemented.

Universal immunization with a tetanus toxoid booster dose is a usual practice in developing countries at this gestation to immunize pregnant patients with tetanus.

At 24–28 weeks

A repeat glucose tolerance test is done at this gestation where the pregnant lady is exposed to the highest carbohydrate intolerance, and optimal glucose metabolism ensures that macrosomia, birth injuries, respiratory distress syndromes, and postnatal hypoglycemic complications of neonates are avoided.

At 32–36 weeks

A fetal well-being scan is done during this time to document optimal fetal growth and placental localization. Strict daily fetal kick count can be explained to the mother as part of antepartum fetal surveillance.

36 weeks to delivery

In cases of previously documented neonatal sepsis with group B streptococcus (GBS), the guidelines from the Centers for Disease Control and Prevention (CDC) advocate GBS screening of pregnant patients and also intrapartum antibiotics for the same [9] (Figure 13.3).

Routine planned termination of pregnancy and labor induction is not advocated until there are specific indications of induction.

Elective cesarean delivery on maternal request should not be encouraged pertaining to the

> Every pregnant woman should undergo screening for group B streptococcus (GBS) at 36 weeks by a high vaginal swab test.
>
> Women with a positive GBS result should be given antibiotic prophylaxis in labor unless they are undergoing elective cesarean.
>
> Women with a negative GBS screen should receive intrapartum antibiotics if they previously gave birth to an infant with GBS-related neonatal sepsis.
>
> Women whose GBS status is unknown should receive intrapartum antibiotics if one or more of the following factors are present:
> Less than 37 weeks' gestation
> Rupture of membranes greater than 18 hours
> Temperature 38°C or higher

Figure 13.3 Overview of maternal group B streptococcus prophylaxis.

apprehension of the mother undergoing the psychological trauma of previous neonatal death. Appropriate counseling and assurance of well-being is of utmost importance.

Labor and postpartum

The neonatologist and the pediatric surgery team, if required, have to be informed prior regarding the scheduled delivery of this mother. Labor and intrapartum fetal monitoring are to be carried out as per the institute protocol. Ensure safe delivery practices and asepsis to avoid neonatal sepsis. Instrumental deliveries are better avoided, but this is up to the treating obstetrician's prerogative.

Neonatal resuscitation and maintaining the asepsis chain following delivery is the next step. Inborn errors of metabolism can be screened with cord blood or by heel prick samples.

Umbilical cord stem cell preservation and cord blood banking is a topic of controversy and can be discussed with the couple prenatally.

ROLE OF UMBILICAL CORD STEM CELL BANKING

Recent evidence-based practices enumerate various benefits of hematopoietic progenitor stem cell preservation for future autologous or allogenic transplantations for multiple oncogenic, immunologic, hematologic, and genetic disorders. A few of them include hemoglobinopathies, childhood malignancies, immunodeficiency syndromes, and bone marrow failure [10].

The added advantage of such cord blood stem cell transplantation is reduced occurrence of graft versus host rejections since the stem cells are not immunologically mature.

A few recommendations are given by the American Academy of Pediatrics (AAP) in their policy statement, for the purposes of parental counseling and decision making [11]:

1. Cord blood preservation does not guarantee future use by the child or family member because the transplanted cells might already contain the genetic inherited mutations of the disease itself. But, there might be some potential benefits of transplantation to an elder sibling with a malignancy or major thalassemia.

2. The paucity of accurate scientific data on autologous stem cell transplantation at the present dictates explanation of the same to the couple and discourages the idea of "biological insurance" to the child.

Ensure rooming-in of the neonate with the mother and initiation of breastfeeding immediately to avail the benefits of colostrum except in suspected inborn errors of metabolism such as galactosemia. Neonatal immunization as per schedule should be practiced.

CONCLUSION

The previous loss of a neonate or an infant automatically confers a state of high-risk pregnancy to the treating obstetrician. With support and a holistic approach in managing such mothers, the results can be a healthy neonate and a favorable pregnancy outcome. Knowledge of the previous neonatal events is vital in the journey of the present pregnancy to avoid unexpected and recurrent mishaps.

REFERENCES

1. Centers for Disease Control and Prevention. Linked Birth/Infant Death Records for 2007–2010 with *ICD-10* codes [Internet]. 2013. Available from: http://wonder.cdc.gov/lbd.html

2. World Health Organization (WHO). *Levels and trends in child mortality 2013*. Geneva, Switzerland: WHO; 2013.

3. Oza S, Lawn JE, Hogan DR, Mathers C, Cousens SN. Neonatal cause-of-death estimates for the early and late neonatal periods for 194 countries: 2000–2013. *Bull World Health Organ*. 2015;93(1):19–28.

4. Roncancio CP, Misnaza SP, Peña IC, Prieto FE, Cannon MJ, Valencia D. Trends and characteristics of fetal and neonatal mortality due to congenital anomalies, Colombia 1999–2008. *J Matern Neonatal Med*. 2018;31(13):1748–55.

5. Knox WE. Sir Archibald Garrod's inborn errors of metabolism. II. Alkaptonuria. *Am J Hum Genet*. 1958;10(2):95–124.

6. Sharma P, Gupta S, Kumar P, Sharma R, Mahapatra TK, Gupta G. *Inborn error of metabolism screening in neonates.* 2019;9(3):196–200.

7. Tsai M-H, Hsu J-F, Chu S-M et al. Incidence, clinical characteristics and risk factors for adverse outcome in neonates with late-onset sepsis. *Pediatr Infect Dis J.* 2014;33(1):e7–13.

8. Brady MT, Polin RA. Prevention and management of infants with suspected or proven neonatal sepsis. *Pediatrics.* 2013; 132:166–8.

9. Pearlman M. Prevention of early-onset group B streptococcal disease in newborns [2] (multiple letters). *Obstet Gynecol.* 2003;102(2):414–5.

10. Jaing TH, Hung IJ, Yang CP, Chen SH, Sun CF, Chow R. Rapid and complete donor chimerism after unrelated mismatched cord blood transplantation in 5 children with β-thalassemia major. *Biol Blood Marrow Transplant.* 2005;11(5):349–53.

11. American Academy of Pediatrics. Cord blood banking for potential future transplantation. *Pediatrics.* 119:2007.

14

Approach to women with a previous child with mental retardation

ASHIMA ARORA AND MINAKSHI ROHILLA

INTRODUCTION

Mental retardation (MR), also referred to as intellectual disability (ID), is defined as a disability characterized by significant limitations in intellectual functioning and adaptive behavior with an onset before the age of 18 years [1]. The definition and classification of MR have been controversial for decades. In easy terms, it is diagnosed when a child demonstrates significantly subaverage general intellectual function, with an overall IQ of less than 70.

The use of the term *mental retardation* is generally limited to older children in whom assessment of IQ is more valid and reliable [2]. The current systems for assessing intelligence are not applicable in younger children, who may therefore be diagnosed with what is commonly termed as *developmental delay*. Developmental delays (DDs) occur due to impairment in the physical, learning, language, or behavior areas. These conditions usually last throughout life and affect day-to-day functioning. DD can be categorized as global developmental delay (GDD) or pervasive developmental delay (PDD). DD that affects all areas of a child's development is generally referred to as GDD, while PDD refers to conditions that involve delay in the development of many basic skills such as the ability to

socialize with others, to communicate, and to use imagination. The term *GDD* is usually reserved for younger children less than 5 years of age.

The overall prevalence of MR worldwide is unknown, and in India it is estimated to be 2%–3% of the total population [3]. Mild MR is almost 10 times more common than moderate or severe MR. The methods of diagnosis of DD/MR and their applicability are a broad topic; this chapter is limited to the approach of an obstetrician to a woman with a previous child with diagnosed DD/MR. The care of the already affected child (both medical and rehabilitative) is beyond the scope of this review.

Classification of mental retardation/developmental delay

Mental retardation has been classified in many ways, most commonly based on severity and etiology. The classification based on severity is presented in Table 14.1.

An IQ greater than 85 is considered normal [4]. This classification based on severity is mainly useful for rehabilitative and prognostication purposes.

Classifying on the basis of etiology, MR can result from a variety of genetic, developmental,

Table 14.1 Classification based on severity of mental retardation (MR)

Grading	IQ (Intelligence Quotient)
Borderline IQ	71–84
Mild MR	50–70
Moderate MR	35–50
Severe MR	20–35
Profound MR	<20

infectious, teratogenic, or traumatic insults to the brain [5]. This trauma may be perinatal or postnatal. The classification based on etiology is as shown in Table 14.2.

IDENTIFICATION OF CAUSE IN A PREVIOUS CHILD

The initial approach to a woman with previous child with MR is to first identify the etiology of MR in that child. It must be realized that the identification of cause of MR may not always be necessary for symptomatic treatment and rehabilitation of the index child and hence must not be forced on all parents. These tests must be offered only if there is a clearly defined purpose for the same. Also, before investing a huge amount of time and money, the

Table 14.2 Classification based on etiology of mental retardation (MR)

Etiology	Prevalence (%)
Chromosomal disorders (*Down syndrome, Prader-Willi syndrome*)	15–40
Nonchromosomal genetic syndromes (*fragile X, tuberous sclerosis, Noonan syndrome*)	6–21
Neurometabolic disorders (*leukodystrophies, mucopolysaccharidosis*)	1–5
Structural central nervous system defects (*microcephaly vera, corpus callosum hypoplasia, Dandy-Walker syndrome*)	2–40
Cerebral palsy–related MR	2.5–23
Environmental insults (*TORCH infections*)	1–25
Idiopathic	30

parents must be counseled that a precise cause will be found in only 50% of cases of moderate to severe MR and an even lesser percentage in mild MR [6].

The American College of Medical Genetics and Genomics, American Academy of Neurology, Practice Committee of the Child Neurology Society, and American Academy of Pediatrics have provided standard guidelines for evaluation of a child with MR/DD. A meticulous detailed history of the affected child's prenatal, perinatal, and postnatal course can offer important clues to the etiology. History should focus on differentiating between a genetic and an acquired cause. A history of exposure to known teratogens like alcohol, premature/traumatic birth, low Apgar scores, and so on, point to acquired causes. Family history of MR, associated congenital malformations, consanguinity, or neonatal death suggest genetic causes. It must be remembered that sometimes, genetic as well as environmental pathogenetic events may contribute to MR in the same individual.

Disease progression must also be noted in detail during history taking. A static course is likely due to teratogenic exposure/traumatic birthing process, while progressive loss of function indicates neurodegenerative or storage disorder. Also, detailed examination of the affected child and parents, in conjunction with imaging and hematologic studies, may lead to identifying the cause.

At the end of history, examination, and investigations, the aim should be to place the affected child in one of the following groups to aid in the management of subsequent pregnancies (Figure 14.1).

ROLE OF OBSTETRICIAN

Out of the many causes of MR, the role of the obstetrician is most important when the suspected etiology is one of the following:

- Genetic
- Related to perinatal events

Role of obstetrician in patients with a previous mentally retarded child due to genetic causes

When the MR is suspected to have some genetic association, the obstetrician must refer the couple to

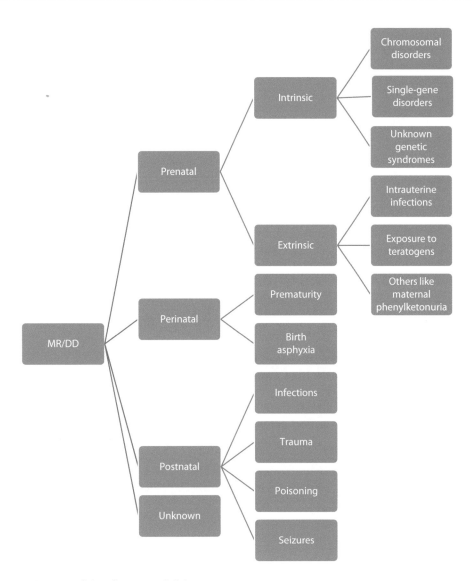

Figure 14.1 Causes of developmental delays.

a genetic counselor in a timely manner for preconceptional counseling. This genetic counselor must:

- Try to assess the accurate diagnosis in a previous child using genetic tests
- Always counsel both parents together
- Provide nondirective counseling, which means that after giving complete impartial information to the couple, they should be left to make a decision

The targeted evaluation based on clinical findings and the latest genomic methods increase the yield of genetic diagnosis. Currently,

array comparative genomic hybridization (aCGH) (microarray) has taken over conventional karyotyping for diagnosing chromosomal abnormalities [7]. The genetic disease must be classified as chromosomal/single-gene disorder/ polygenic/multifactorial or epigenetic based on test results, and further counseling should proceed accordingly.

The roles of genetic counselor are multifactorial and mainly include the following:

- If the cause is found to be sporadic, the couple must be reassured that the risk of recurrence is not more than the general population.

- For familial genetic defects, the couple must be educated about the pattern of inheritance and the chances of recurrence of disease in their offspring.
- The couple must be provided detailed information about the prenatal diagnostic tests available for their disorder in the subsequent pregnancies, and their feasibility, availability, and cost.
- The couple must be encouraged to make an informed choice about future reproduction in cases of severe dysfunction with known recurrence.

The obstetrician must collaborate with the geneticist regarding the prenatal diagnostic tests that need to be performed in the next pregnancy of the couple with mentally retarded child.

Role of obstetrician in patients with a previous mentally retarded child due to perinatal events

Mental retardation can be secondary to perinatal asphyxia, which is defined as a lack of blood flow or gas exchange to or from the fetus immediately before, during, or after birth. The incidence of significant perinatal asphyxia is highly variable in different parts of the world depending on the care received by pregnant women, ranging from 2 per 1000 births in the developed world to 2 per 100 in developing countries where access to maternal care is limited. This perinatal/birth asphyxia leads to profound neurological sequelae in more than 25% of the affected babies [8]. The majority of cases of birth asphyxia occur intrapartum, although around 20% of cases are antepartum, while rarely, early postnatal events may also contribute to it. Therefore, thorough history of the previous pregnancy that resulted in mental retardation is mandatory for the obstetrician managing the present pregnancy, with special focus on birthing history. History of birth trauma, difficult instrumental delivery, macrosomia, difficult breech delivery, and so on, must be elicited. Also, maternal complications, such as hypertensive disorders of pregnancy, that may lead to placental insufficiency or preterm births leading to developmental delay in the neonate must be asked about. Overall, the most likely cause of perinatal asphyxia must be ascertained. Some causes such as perinatal infections are known not to recur, while others such as untreated Rh iso-immunization may result in cognitive delays, deafness, and cerebral palsy in survivors.

The mode and gestation of delivery need to be individualized. There are no recommendations to perform elective cesarean section in women with previous history of birth asphyxia. However, every attempt needs to be made to ensure good perinatal outcome. A population-based cohort study conducted in the Netherlands over a span of 9 years involving approximately 200,000 women concluded that if the first-born child of a woman had evidence of birth asphyxia, then the risk of recurrence of birth asphyxia in subsequent delivery was the same as the general nulliparous population. However, this risk was halved in women who had no evidence of birth asphyxia in their first childbirth [9].

DOWN SYNDROME

The most common form of inherited intellectual disability is Down syndrome, with a prevalence of 1 in 800 live births [10]. The clinical presentation of Down syndrome (DS) may vary significantly, and though the diagnosis can be made prenatally, prenatal assessment cannot predict the severity of complications in an affected DS fetus. Almost half of the fetuses with DS do not survive pregnancy, ending in early-trimester loss or stillbirth.

Approximately 95% of cases of DS result from nondisjunction involving chromosome 21, while the remaining cases result from translocations or somatic mosaicism [11]. As DS is the most common single diagnosis of MR in children with prenatal diagnosis possible in most cases, offering screening for aneuploidy during pregnancy is the standard of care and must be done in all women at the first prenatal visit. The woman must be informed about the prenatal screening and diagnostic tests available for aneuploidy, and each individual patient may decide her own test based on age, reproductive history, family history, finances, personal desire for informational accuracy, and so on.

Salient features for screening and diagnosis of Down syndrome

1. Every antenatal woman should have the choice to undergo screening tests, diagnostic tests, or no testing for aneuploidy based on her informed autonomous decision.
2. The types of screening methods available are
   - Single screening tests (dual, triple, quadruple, penta screen)
   - Combined first- and second-trimester screening (integrated and sequential screening) (Table 14.3) [13]
   - Ultrasonographic screening
   - Cell-free DNA screening modality (cfDNA), commonly called noninvasive prenatal testing (NIPT)
3. As a screening modality, either first-trimester combined serum screening with nuchal translucency (NT) or cfDNA may be used. Both tests have different limitations and strengths—no one test is superior to another. Other serum screening tests such as triple screen and quadruple screen have lower sensitivity.
4. Both screening tests (first-trimester combined screen and cfDNA) should not be done concurrently in the same woman.
5. cfDNA should not be done as a follow-up for abnormal serum screening. An abnormal screening test must be followed up by a diagnostic test that can diagnose/exclude aneuploidy. Also, patients with positive serum screens are at risk for other aneuploidies or adverse outcomes, and performing cfDNA in these women may delay time to definitive diagnosis or provide false reassurance.
6. Screening with cfDNA can be performed at any gestation from 10 weeks onward up to term. It offers the highest reported detection rate for Down syndrome among all screening tests—more than 98% detection. The detection rate is lower for trisomy 13 and trisomy 18. However, women with low fetal fraction (less than 4%) who have no reportable results must be directly counseled for diagnostic testing, as these women have an increased risk for fetal aneuploidy.
7. A second-trimester ultrasonography must not be used alone to diagnose or exclude DS because it detects only 50%–60% of cases. Each ultrasonographic soft marker has its own likelihood ratio for DS and must be considered in conjunction with serum screening results if available. The soft markers with the highest likelihood ratio for DS are increased NT and cystic hygroma in the first trimester and mild ventriculomegaly and

Table 14.3 Types of screening for risk of aneuploidy

1. *Integrated screening*
   Final result reported after completion of both first- and second-trimester screens
   a. Positive: Offer diagnostic test
   b. Negative: No further testing required
2. *Stepwise sequential*
   First-trimester test results
   a. Positive: Offer diagnostic test
   b. Negative: Offer second-trimester screening (quadruple screen)
   c. Final: Final risk assessment based on first- and second-trimester results
3. *Contingent sequential*
   First-trimester test results
   a. Positive: Offer diagnostic test
   b. Negative: No further testing required
   c. Intermediate: Offer second-trimester screening
   d. Final: Final risk assessment based on first- and second-trimester results

increased nuchal fold thickness in the second trimester.

8. Any risk factor for aneuploidy including abnormal serum screen results, abnormal or "no call" cfDNA, or ultrasound abnormalities with high likelihood ratios should result in detailed counseling and offering diagnostic testing.

9. In case an invasive diagnostic test is performed during pregnancy, the tissue must be sent for microarray. Microarray has many advantages over conventional karyotype including the ability to detect deletions and microduplications, which can be missed on conventional karyotype. In fetuses with structural anomalies on ultrasound, the difference in detection rates of microarray and karyotype is even more pronounced. It may be reasonable to start with a conventional karyotype if there is a very high suspicion of common aneuploidy [12].

Summary of risk assessment with first-trimester combined screen

The conventional or traditional screening tests include measurement of multiple serum markers or analytes that are then converted to a multiple of the median (MoM) value by adjusting for gestational age, maternal age, maternal weight, race, ethnicity, diabetes, number of fetuses with chorionicity, and type of pregnancy (*in vitro* fertilization). This allows for comparison of the results from different laboratories and populations (Tables 14.4 and 14.5) [14]. This analyte-based screening result is based on composite likelihood ratios and therefore provides specific risks for aneuploidies as ratios that represent the positive predictive value (Figure 14.2).

Table 14.4 Serum β-human chorionic gonadotropin (hCG) and pregnancy-associated plasma protein-A (PAPP-A) levels in first-trimester screening

Karyotype	β-hCG multiple of the median	PAPP-A multiple of the median
Normal	1.0	1.0
Trisomy 21	>2.0	<0.5
Trisomy 18	<0.2	<0.2
Trisomy 13	<0.5	<0.3

Table 14.5 Second-trimester serum screening in Down syndrome

β-human chorionic gonadotropin (hCG)	>2.0 multiple of the median (MoM)
Inhibin A	>1.77 MoM
α-fetoprotein	Reduced by 25%
Free estriol	Reduced by 25%

CONCLUSION

Worldwide, up to 20% of children suffer from debilitating mental illness. Parents of such children face unique psychological, emotional, and social challenges. Therefore, the obstetrician managing the subsequent pregnancies needs to be well acquainted with the needs of the couple. Adequate knowledge about the causes, a team approach with a geneticist and a neonatologist, and an attitude of compassion can lead to desirable outcomes in subsequent pregnancies in most cases.

POINTS TO PONDER

- MR/DD is defined as an IQ less than 70.
- MR can result from a variety of genetic, developmental, infectious, teratogenic, or traumatic insults to the brain. These insults may be prenatal, perinatal, or postnatal. More than one factor may coexist in one patient.
- The initial approach of an obstetrician to a woman with previous child with MR who is planning subsequent pregnancy is to first identify the etiology of MR in the affected child.
- If the cause is suspected to be genetic, detailed preconceptional counseling must be offered to the couple. The geneticist can guide the couple to plan detailed genetic tests of the affected child and prenatal diagnostic tests in further pregnancies.
- MR secondary to birth asphyxia is usually nonrecurring.
- Down syndrome is the most common inherited form of ID; therefore, every antenatal woman must be offered aneuploidy screening in pregnancy.

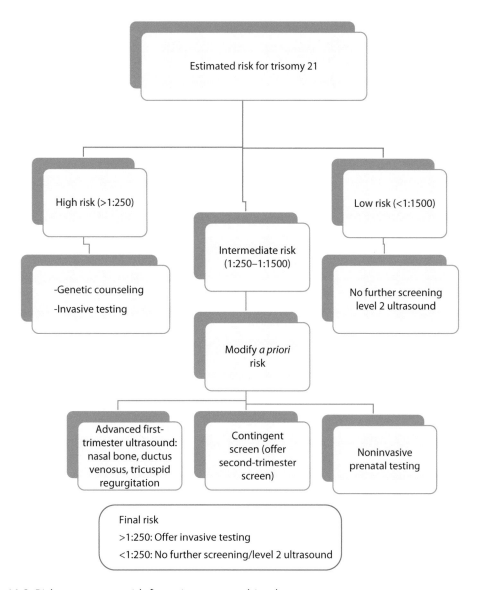

Figure 14.2 Risk assessment with first-trimester combined screen.

REFERENCES

1. *American Psychiatric Association: Task Force on DSM-IV. Diagnostic and Statistical Manual of Mental Disorders: DSM-IV*. Washington, DC: American Psychiatric Association; 1994.

2. American Academy of Pediatrics Committee on Children with Disabilities. Developmental surveillance and screening in infants and young children. *Pediatrics*. 2001;108:192–6.

3. Kabra M, Gulati S. Mental retardation. *Indian J Pediatr*. 2003;70:153–8.

4. Battaglia A, Carey JC. Diagnostic evaluation of developmental delay/mental retardation: An overview. *Am J Med Genet C Semin Med Genet*. 2003;117C:3–14.

5. Aggarwal S, Bogula VR, Mandal K, Kumar R, Phadke SR. Aetiologic spectrum of mental retardation and development delay in India. *Indian J Med Res*. 2012;136: 436–44.

6. Curry CJ, Stevenson RE, Aughton D et al. Evaluation of mental retardation: Recommendations of a Consensus Conference:

American College of Medical Genetics. *Am J Med Genet.* 1997;72:468–77.

7. Wapner RJ, Martin CL, Levy B et al. Chromosomal microarray versus karyotyping for prenatal diagnosis. *N Engl J Med.* 2012;367:2175–84.

8. Martin JA, Hamilton BE, Ventura SJ, Osterman MJ, Mathews TJ. Births: Final data for 2011. *Natl Vital Stat Rep.* 2013;62:1–70.

9. Ensing S, Schaaf JM, Abu-Hanna A, Mol BWJ, Ravelli ACJ. Recurrence risk of low Apgar score among term singletons: A population-based cohort study. *Acta Obstet Gynecol Scand.* 2014;93:897–904.

10. Nussbaum RL, McInnes RR, Willard HF. *Principles of Clinical Cytogenetics and Genome Analysis. Thompson & Thompson Genetics in Medicine.* Philadelphia, PA: Elsevier; 2016:57–74.

11. Sherman SL, Allen EG, Bean LH, Freeman SB. Epidemiology of Down syndrome. *Ment Retard Dev Disabil Res Rev.* 2007;13:221–7.

12. American College of Obstetricians and Gynecologists. Screening for fetal aneuploidy. Practice Bulletin No. 163. *Obstet Gynecol.* 2016;127:e123–37.

13. Gabbe S. *Obstetrics: Normal and Problem Pregnancies.* 7th ed. Philadelphia, PA: Elsevier; 2017.

14. Arias F. *Arias' Practical Guide to High-Risk Pregnancy and Delivery.* Philadelphia, PA: Elsevier Health Sciences APAC; 2015.

15

Approach to women with a previous child with a genetic disorder

SURBHI GUPTA

INTRODUCTION

Worldwide there is a demographic transition from a decrease in communicable diseases to a relative increase in noncommunicable diseases. Congenital anomalies are one such group of noncommunicable diseases that have become an important cause of mortality, especially in the perinatal period. Congenital anomalies are functional or structural defects occurring mostly during intrauterine life and can be identified before birth, at birth, or later in life. The Global Burden of Disease Study 2013 identified congenital anomalies among the top 10 causes of mortality in children less than 5 years of age [1]. According to the March of Dimes (MOD) Global Report on Birth Defects, worldwide 7.9 million births occur annually with serious birth defects, and 94% of these births occur in middle- and low-income countries [2].

Many congenital anomalies are due to defects in the gene or chromosome. These types of disorders are called *genetic disorders*. A genetic disorder is a cause of perinatal mortality in 20%–25% of cases [3]. The defect can range from a single base in the DNA to an entire chromosomal abnormality involving the subtraction or addition of an entire

chromosome or set of chromosomes. Some of these disorders are inherited, while others are due to acquired changes in a gene. There are many factors that influence the prevalence of genetic disorders in India. First, consanguineous marriages are common in many communities in India. Second, India has a very high birth rate. Therefore, large numbers of babies are born with genetic disorders. Third, better diagnostic facilities and medical care have led to the early identification of genetic diseases.

There are many tests available to assess the risk of having a child with genetic disorders. These tests are called *screening tests*. Other tests available are called *diagnostic tests*, which can accurately detect any specific problems in the baby. Both of these tests are offered to a pregnant woman. A couple with a previous child with genetic disorder should undergo counseling by a geneticist and then decide on testing.

HUMAN GENES

It is worth understanding the human genome first before discussing genetic disorders. The human genome is the entire "treasury of human inheritance." It consists of 46 chromosomes, including

44 autosomal chromosomes and 2 sex chromosomes. These chromosomes are made up of DNA base pairs. A short segment of DNA forms a gene. Genes contain the instruction manual for our bodies. They direct the building of all proteins that make our body function. Genes are present in pairs, except those on sex chromosomes. After fertilization, the embryo contains 23 pairs of chromosomes (one pair from each parent). Therefore, a baby receives half of its genes from the mother and the other half from the father.

MODES OF INHERITANCE

Different types of genetic inheritance are as follows:

1. Single-gene genetic inheritance
2. Multifactorial genetic inheritance
3. Chromosomal abnormalities
4. Mitochondrial genetic inheritance

1. Single-gene genetic inheritance

Single-gene inheritance is also called Mendelian or monogenetic inheritance. This is caused by changes or mutations that occur in the DNA sequence of a single gene. Single-gene disorders are inherited in patterns that can be recognized: autosomal dominant, autosomal recessive, and sex-linked.

- *Autosomal dominant*: Only one copy of the disease allele is necessary for an individual to be susceptible to expressing the phenotype. The disease allele is located on any of the 44 autosomal chromosomes. If one parent is affected, then there is a 50% chance that the offspring will inherit the disease. Examples include neurofibromatosis type 1, Marfan syndrome, and Huntington's chorea.
- *Autosomal recessive*: Two copies of a disease allele are required for an individual to be susceptible to expressing the phenotype. Therefore, parents are carriers in the majority of diseases and are asymptomatic. The child will only be affected when he or she inherits two abnormal copies of the gene; hence, there is a 25% probability that the child will have the disorder. Similar to the carrier parents, there is a 50% probability that the child will be a carrier of the disorder. Some recessive disorders are known to occur more often in certain races and ethnic

groups, for example, cystic fibrosis, sickle cell anemia, and Tay-Sachs disease.
- *Sex-linked disorders*: Disorders that are caused by genes located on the sex chromosomes (X or Y chromosome) are referred to as sex-linked disorders. These include X-linked recessive and X-linked dominant.
  - *X-linked recessive*: Females are not usually affected as they have two X chromosomes. For a carrier female, there is a 50% chance that her son will inherit the disease and a 50% chance her daughter will be a carrier. For an affected female, all of her daughters will be unaffected carriers and all of her sons will be affected. Affected males transmit the disease allele to all of their daughters but not to their sons. Examples include Duchenne muscular dystrophy and fragile X syndrome.
  - *X-linked dominant*: A few diseases may be so severe in affected boys that the pregnancy miscarries prior to disease recognition; therefore, only affected girls are born with the disease. Examples include Aicardi syndrome and Rett syndrome.

2. Multifactorial genetic inheritance

Disorders caused by environmental factors leading to mutations in various genes are multifactorial genetic disorders. These disorders can run in families, but the ways in which they are inherited are not completely understood. Neural tube defects, heart defects, and cleft palate are examples of multifactorial disorders. Many people are born with genes that give them a higher chance of developing cancer or diabetes mellitus but never develop these diseases. This may be because an environmental factor, such as exposure to a cancer-causing chemical, smoking, a high-fat diet, or being overweight, is needed to trigger the disease.

3. Chromosomal abnormalities

- *Aneuploidy*: Some genetic disorders are caused by having too many or too few chromosomes. Having an abnormal number of chromosomes is called *aneuploidy*. Aneuploidy usually occurs because the egg or the sperm contains an abnormal number of chromosomes. These errors occur when the eggs or sperm are formed and usually happen by chance. However, the chance of these errors occurring in a woman's eggs increases as she ages. The chance of aneuploidy therefore increases as well. Most children with aneuploidy have intellectual disabilities and/or physical defects. The most common type of aneuploidy is a trisomy, which is caused because of an extra chromosome. Examples of trisomies include trisomy 13 (Patau syndrome), trisomy 18 (Edwards syndrome), and trisomy 21 (Down syndrome).

In comparison to trisomy, a monosomy is caused because of a missing chromosome. Monosomies are much rarer than trisomies. An example of a monosomy is Turner syndrome, where a female has only one X chromosome.

- *Structural chromosomal disorders*: Some genetic diseases are caused by problems with the structure of chromosomes. These disorders are sometimes called *structural chromosomal disorders*. Some structural chromosomal disorders are inherited due to the presence of abnormal chromosomes in the eggs or sperm. Others occur during prenatal development or even later in life.

In these types of disorders, a part/piece of a chromosome can be missing (deletion), a part/piece of a chromosome can be duplicated (duplication), or a piece of a chromosome can break off and relocate to another chromosome (translocation).

Translocations do not always cause a disease or physical disability. A translocation is called unbalanced when genetic material is lost or gained. A balanced translocation does not result in any gain or loss of genetic material.

People who have a balanced translocation usually have no medical effects.

However, a person with a balanced translocation can have a child with an unbalanced translocation. Unbalanced translocations also have been linked to repeated miscarriages.

Structural chromosomal disorders are named according to the chromosome number that is affected and sometimes by the location where the deletion, insertion, or translocation occurs. Examples of structural chromosomal disorders include 5p deletion syndrome (cri-du-chat syndrome) and 22q11.2 deletion syndrome (DiGeorge syndrome).

4. Mitochondrial genetic inheritance

Only females can transmit the trait to the offspring. An affected female will transmit the disease to male and female children alike. A mother with a small number of mitochondrial DNA mutated will be unaffected. If the mitochondria with mutated DNA replicate more in the zygote, the baby will be affected. Hence, disease status depends on mutated mitochondrial DNA load. Examples of mitochondrial disease include Leber hereditary optic neuropathy and MELAS (mitochondrial myopathy, encephalopathy, lactic acidosis, and stroke).

RISK FACTORS

The option of preconception or early pregnancy assistance is considered, and the couple reaches out to a primary care group for a range of reasons. The probability of birth of a child with a genetic disorder escalates with the following risk factors:

- Older age in either the father or mother [4]
- Presence of a genetic disorder in one or both parents
- Another child with a genetic disease was born to this couple
- A strong family history of a certain genetic disease exists
- Either or both parents come from an ethnic background that has an excessive rate of carriers of particular genetic conditions

The key role of every member of the primary care group is to look for the mentioned risk elements and refer such a couple to a genetic counselor. A counselor who specializes in genetic disorders or any alternate health wellness provider with proficiency in genetics should be useful in the previously mentioned situations. A genetic counselor can study the family health history and make recommendations about which tests are most appropriate for the couple. The procedure involves two steps:

1. Find and compute the risk
2. Assess options, given the genetic threats

IDENTIFYING THE RISK

Genetic counseling is a two-way interaction and not merely advice giving. It is a process that occurs over a period of time. The client's autonomy in decision making varies depending on personal, familial, and cultural contexts. It should help people cope with reproductive and other implications of that disorder.

We discuss the case of a couple with a baby with a genetic disorder. It is preferable if the couple asks for help in the prepregnancy period. There is ample time to clinically evaluate the condition, conduct baseline tests, provide cross-consultation if required, arrive at a diagnosis, and have the results in hand. Proper planning and monitoring of the subsequent pregnancy can be done. Workup begins with an evaluation of the child with a genetic disorder (Figure 15.1).

Step 1: History taking

Drawing up a pedigree chart by the process of detailing the family's past is the mandatory first step of a genetic consultation. The process should thoroughly ask both individuals in the couple about any medical records of all previous children and other family members such as parents, brothers, and sisters, and maternal and paternal uncles/aunts/grandparents. Observations from each of the questions should be noted in detail, and wherever relevant and necessary, check the age and cause of death. Even if it is discovered that the disorder relates to one partner's family, it is critical to obtain details about the other partner's family. It is important to keep in mind the ethnic background and place of birth as they may have a part to play in considering the risks

of recessive conditions. The care team should refer to the reports of the family for all relevant medical history. Review photographs of affected family members, if available. The couple should be asked specific questions, such as were there any ultrasonography findings during the prenatal examination (e.g., increased nuchal translucency, congenital heart defect, or cleft lip/palate); is there a history of exposure to teratogen; what is the birth, developmental, and growth history of the child; what was the age of onset and nature of progression of the problem.

Step 2: Examination

A detailed head-to-toe examination of the affected child should be done. Look for any dysmorphic features. This should be followed by a detailed systemic examination. After receiving informed consent from the parents, photographs of the child should be taken.

Step 3: Perform test

Previous child is alive

Yes	Test for chromosomal abnormalities
	Test for single-gene defect
No	Carrier screening
	Prenatal diagnosis

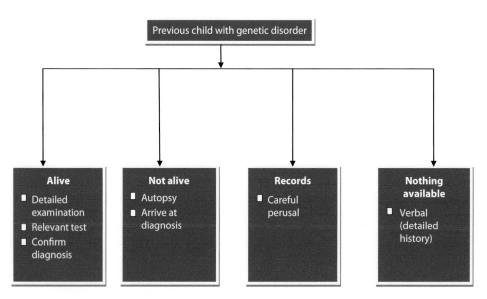

Figure 15.1 Evaluation of a child with a genetic disorder.

TESTS FOR CHROMOSOMAL ABNORMALITIES

1. Karyotype by conventional chromosomal analysis
2. Fluorescence *in situ* hybridization
3. Multiplex ligation-dependent probe amplification
4. Prenatal bacterial artificial chromosomes on beads
5. Comparative genomic hybridization

1. Karyotype by conventional chromosomal analysis

In order to detect the absent, additional, or damaged chromosomes, taking a picture of the chromosomes and ordering them from smallest to largest is done. This is called a *karyotype*. Conventionally, a magnification of about 1000 at metaphase is needed to perform microscopic studies of chromosomes. At the metaphase stage, the visual karyotype is prepared by arresting the dividing cells with a microtubule polymerization inhibitor such as colchicines and then is followed up with cells spread on a glass slide and stained with Giemsa staining (G banding). A karyotype can show if:

- The number of chromosomes is abnormal.
- The shape of one or more chromosomes is abnormal.
- A chromosome is broken.

The major disadvantage is that it takes approximately 2 weeks to perform and cannot identify small chromosomal abnormalities.

2. Fluorescence *in situ* hybridization

A chromosome sample is denatured on a glass slide so that the DNA is single stranded and then mixed with a fluorescent DNA probe. This is a sequence of DNA that is complementary to the sequence of interest. The sequence-specific hybridization is formed by the overnight incubation. If a chromosomal preparation shows only one signal, then there is a deletion of the second copy of DNA sequence; if there are more than two signals, then duplication is present. Fluorescence *in situ* hybridization (FISH) can identify only a known microdeletion syndrome and therefore it

is only used to confirm a specific diagnosis suspected from clinical features.

3. Multiplex ligation-dependent probe amplification

This technique can identify many more abnormalities in one reaction than can be identified by FISH, but it is still limited to the most common deletion and microdeletion syndromes. Forty probes can be used per experiment [5].

4. Prenatal bacterial artificial chromosomes on beads

This test identifies common trisomies 13, 18, 21, and X/Y and nine other common microdeletion syndromes. A bacterial artificial chromosome is a sequence of DNA that has been incorporated into a bacterium to allow a large amount of the sequence of interest to be manufactured. Bacterial artificial chromosomes derived from each chromosomal region of interest are then immobilized on a bead, which then has three fluorochromes attached for quantifying the reaction. The sample DNA is then added and analyzed. It uses two probes per chromosome arm and three for each acrocentric chromosome and has been shown to be an accurate method of identifying trisomies [6]. As culture failure is not an issue, this test can be used on products of conception. Terminal duplication and deletion have a lower overall pickup rate and may not be suitable for this analysis.

5. Comparative genomic hybridization

The basis of this test is comparison of total genomic DNA of the given sample DNA (e.g., tumor DNA) to genomic DNA of a normal cell. The glass slide onto which thousands of short sequences of DNA (probes) are noticed is known as an *array*. The patient's DNA is labeled with fluorescent dye and the control sample with another colored dye. The patient and control samples are denatured to become single stranded and then mixed together and applied to the slide. Hybridization occurs where the patient's DNA joins the matching probes on the array. The array is then scanned to measure the intensity of each dye. Comparative genomic hybridization is now the investigation of choice for a developmentally delayed child without an obvious diagnosis. It identifies the underlying cause of mental retardation in an additional 12%–15% of children without a previous diagnosis [7]. The disadvantage of the test is that it may identify variations in quantity of DNA that are of unknown significance.

TESTS FOR SINGLE-GENE DEFECTS

A gene is divided into exons and introns; the coding regions are the exons, and these need to be sequenced along with either side of the exon/intron boundaries. Tests for single-gene defects include the following:

1. Sanger sequencing
2. Amplification refractory mutation system test
3. Next-generation sequencing

1. Sanger sequencing

This requires that double-stranded DNA be denatured, normal nucleotides and altered nucleotides labeled with a fluorescent dye, and a polymerase then added and run on a sequence. It is excellent for sequencing accurately for diseases like sickle cell anemia with known mutation. The problem with this technique is that only a small amount of DNA can be analyzed in any reaction, which makes the technique slow and expensive.

2. Amplification refractory mutation system test

In this test, for each mutation that is examined, there will be two reactions. The normal sequence will only amplify the normal, and the abnormal will only amplify the abnormal. This is a rapid method for looking for common mutations as seen in cystic fibrosis or thalassemia. It is only suitable for single base changes or small deletions [8].

3. Next-generation sequencing

This technique involves fragmentation of the whole genome. The areas of interest are then pulled down onto a slide that consists of DNA probes. The rest of the unwanted DNA is washed off the sample. The sample DNA is then amplified

and read by a number of different platforms. The accuracy of the test depends on how many copies of each region of interest are captured, known as the depth of the read. Having sequenced multiple genes, the data need to be analyzed, a large number of variants are identified, and then it is necessary to identify which variant, if any, is likely to be pathologic [9]. It allows large amounts of DNA to be sequenced at the same time. If there is a distinctive phenotype, then comparing affected children for mutations within the same gene is a very powerful way to identify the underlying genetic cause of the phenotype. This technique is extremely useful for diseases such as Noonan syndrome, which has a phenotype that can be caused by multiple different genes.

CARRIER SCREENING

Both father and mother are subjected to carrier screening to determine if a person has a gene for any recessive disorder. For this test, options available are to use a sample of blood or a sample of saliva for study in a laboratory. Tests performed on the sample can determine whether the person carries the specific genes. Carrier screening has traditionally been recommended for people who are at higher risk of certain genetic disorders because of their family history, ethnicity, or race.

Another carrier screening option is called *expanded carrier screening*. It is now possible with new technology to screen for a wide variety of disorders with a high degree of accuracy and at a relatively low cost. It is better suited for those who do not have a previously known family history. Many laboratories now offer expanded carrier screening. Once you know your carrier status for a disorder, you do not need to be tested again in a future pregnancy for that disorder.

Results

In the event of a negative test result, then no further steps are needed; if the result is positive, then the other partner is subjected to the test. If a subsequent test of the other partner is also positive, then the risks of having a child with the disorder along with the other options are to be explained by the genetic counselor or a health-care provider. Genetic counseling is crucial for recognizing the genetic risk, referring patients appropriately, and informing patients about genetic issues that are relevant to decision making [10].

Timing

Carrier screening can be done either before pregnancy or during the early weeks of pregnancy.

If either partner is a disease carrier

Being a carrier does not usually affect the person's own health. It also does not mean that all their children will be affected. The health-care provider or genetic counselor can calculate the chances that a baby will possess the disorder or be a potential carrier. In such scenarios, the couple can think about several options as follows:

- If done before pregnancy, then the couple may opt to continue with becoming pregnant with the option of considering prenatal diagnostic testing. They may choose to use *in vitro* fertilization with donor eggs or sperm to achieve pregnancy. Preimplantation genetic diagnosis can be used with this option.
- If already pregnant, then they may choose to have diagnostic testing, if it is available, to see if the baby will be born with the disorder. The couple should consider telling other family members if they are carriers. They may be at risk of being carriers themselves.

PRENATAL TESTS

- Screening tests
- Diagnostic tests

Screening tests

The risk that a baby will have Down syndrome and other trisomies as well as neural tube defects is assessed using these parental screening tests. The tests help to assess the risk of the baby having these disorders and not if the baby actually has these disorders. The screening tests are very safe and do not have any risks for the unborn baby.

These tests can be performed in the first or second trimester. Results of these tests can also be combined in various ways; integrated or sequential screening has a higher detection rate than tests performed independently.

The gestational age and the team's assessment of which test is best for the couple determine what types of screening tests are to be performed.

Women who are at high risk of having a child with aneuploidy may be offered another type of test that is known as the cell-free DNA test.

CELL-FREE DNA TEST

The cell-free DNA test is a screening test available for women. A tiny amount of fetal DNA, which comes mainly from the placenta, circulates in the mother's blood. The mother's blood is taken as a sample to assess various trisomies and sex chromosome abnormalities [11]. The test is 99% correct in spotting cases of Down syndrome and has a very low rate of false-positive results for females who are at escalated risk of having a baby with a chromosomal disorder. A female can be subjected to this test as early as the 10th week of pregnancy. Results take approximately 1 week to process.

The cell-free DNA test is a screening test best suited for women who have an escalated risk of having a child with a genetic disorder, such as women who already have a baby with a chromosomal disorder. This process has certain limitations. Any female carrying more than one baby is advised against undergoing this test. Second, it does not inspect for neural tube defects. To detect these disorders, an additional screening test is necessary. Also, although it is highly accurate in identifying chromosomal issues in high-risk women, it is not as accurate as diagnostic tests. Hence, it is advised to follow up a positive test result with a diagnostic test.

FIRST-TRIMESTER SCREENING

A maternal age and blood test combined with an ultrasound examination are part of first-trimester screening. This is called *combined first-trimester screening*. It is done near the 11-week (13+6 weeks) period of gestation to gauge the risk of trisomy 21 and other aneuploidies. The mother's blood is tested to measure the levels of two different proteins (β-human chorionic gonadotropin [β-hCG] and pregnancy-associated plasma protein-A [PAPP-A]). An ultrasound examination, called *nuchal translucency screening*, is used to measure the thickness at the back of the neck of the baby.

An escalation in the thickness acts as a marker for Down syndrome, trisomy 18, or other problems.

SECOND-TRIMESTER SCREENING

There are three main tests used in screening for chromosomal abnormalities in the second trimester, namely, detailed ultrasound, the triple test, and the quadruple test.

The biochemical markers used in the triple test are α-fetoprotein, β-hCG, and free estriol. The quadruple test adds inhibin A.

Comprehensive ultrasound, sometimes referred to as detailed anomaly scan, is carried out between 18 and 20 weeks of gestation. It is not the first choice to screen for chromosomal abnormalities but can be used to screen for trisomy 21 and other chromosomal abnormalities for women who first present at this stage.

There are many markers that can be seen at this ultrasound, called *soft markers*, e.g., increased nuchal fold thickness, echogenic bowel, foci in heart, short humerus or femur, cleft lip, and many more. However, the presence of these soft markers does not necessarily indicate a chromosomal anomaly but merely indicates an increased risk.

The triple test and the quadruple test have become less popular as the accuracy of first-trimester screening has improved.

RESULTS

It is critical to be aware of the chances of false-positive and false-negative results and the consequences of these results with any type of testing.

Results may also be described as "screen negative" or "screen positive" depending on whether the risk is lower or higher than the cutoff point. Different laboratories have different cutoff points for what is considered screen positive and screen negative.

IF SCREENING TEST RESULTS SHOW AN INCREASED RISK

If the results of a screening test show an escalated risk, then further evaluation by diagnostic testing should be done.

Diagnostic tests

Whether the baby has a genetic condition or not can be assessed with the information provided by diagnostic tests. These tests are done on DNA obtained from fetal cells. The tests can be done as early as from 11 to 13 weeks of gestation via chorionic villus sampling (CVS) or from 15 to 20 weeks via amniocentesis [12]. The result is generated within 7 or 15 days, respectively [12]. Different techniques exist to analyze the cells. Once the cells are obtained, they can be studied in different ways depending on the disorders being tested for. One need is to test for monogenic diseases. If the mutations are known, then the disease can be tested for by direct mutation analysis and if not known, then by linkage analysis [13]. A specific analysis test is always accompanied by paternity verification and analysis for contamination [13].

AMNIOCENTESIS

To perform amniocentesis, a sample of amniotic fluid is extracted by means of a thin needle that is steered through the woman's abdomen and uterus.

Amniotic fluid contains cells from the unborn child. These cells then are referred to a laboratory, where they are grown in a special culture. When the cells are ready, they are analyzed to determine whether the baby has certain disorders, such as trisomy 21 or any specific genetic disorders conditional to family history and ultrasound exam observations.

The amniotic fluid can also be tested to detect neural tube defects.

Issues like cramping, vaginal bleeding, infection, and leaking of amniotic fluid may occur due to complications of amniocentesis.

CHORIONIC VILLUS SAMPLING

CVS is generally performed earlier than amniocentesis. This earlier time frame allows more time to think about options and to make decisions. However, CVS is not as commonly performed as amniocentesis and may not be accessible at all hospitals or health centers. It is important to note that CVS should be performed by an experienced health-care provider.

A tiny sample of tissue is taken from the placenta to perform CVS. The same genetic makeup of the child can be found in the cells on the tissue. To obtain the sample, a small tube can be inserted through the woman's vagina and cervix (transcervical CVS) or a thin needle can be inserted through the abdomen and wall of the uterus (transabdominal CVS).

As usual, the cells are grown in a culture after being sent to a laboratory and are then subsequently analyzed.

Vaginal bleeding, leakage of amniotic fluid, and infection are some of the complications from CVS. The risk of miscarriage with CVS is similar to amniocentesis so should be performed by an experienced person in a well-suited center.

PREIMPLANTATION GENETIC DIAGNOSIS

Couples using *in vitro* fertilization for conception may be subjected to preimplantation genetic diagnosis if they are at an escalated risk of having a child with a genetic disorder. An embryo is tested to determine if it has a specific known genetic disorder for which the couple is at risk, before transferring it to a woman's uterus. A genome-wide protocol using next-generation sequencing has been tested for the identification of family mutations together with cytogenetic screening in embryo biopsies [14–16].

CONCLUSION

A variety of causes exist for a couple to be exposed to escalated genetic risk. It is important for the geneticist as well as the primary care team members to ensure that the facts are well established, relevant tests are done, and the final diagnosis is made.

The next step after the diagnosis is the counseling process that will help the individual or family to:

1. Understand the disease, its diagnosis, its course in the human body, available treatment and further management
2. Gain knowledge about the type of inheritance of the disease and its chances of recurrence
3. Comprehend the options available for dealing with the risk of recurrence
4. Take the best possible path that appears to be appropriate in view of their risk and, simultaneously, in accordance with their ethical and religious standards
5. Take the necessary steps to deal with the disorder

REFERENCES

1. Global Burden of Disease Pediatrics Collaboration. Global and national burden of diseases and injuries among children and adolescents between 1990 and 2013: Findings from the Global Burden of Disease 2013 study. *JAMA Pediatr.* 2016;170(3):267–87.
2. Christianson A, Howson CP, Modell B. March of Dimes: Global report on birth defects, the hidden toll of dying and disabled children. Research report. White Plains, NY: March of Dimes Birth Defects Foundation; 2006.
3. Stavljenić-Rukavina A. Prenatal diagnosis of chromosomal disorders-molecular aspects. *EJIFCC.* 2008;19(1):2.
4. Allen EG, Freeman SB, Druschel C et al. Maternal age and risk for trisomy 21 assessed by the origin of chromosome nondisjunction: A report from the Atlanta and National Down Syndrome Projects. *Hum Genet.* 2009;125(1):41–52.
5. Willis AS, van den Veyver I, Eng CM. Multiplex ligation-dependent probe amplification (MLPA) and prenatal diagnosis. *Prenat Diagn.* 2012;32(4):315–20.
6. Grati FR, Gomes DM, Ganesamoorthy D et al. Application of a new molecular technique for the genetic evaluation of products of conception. *Prenat Diagn.* 2013;33(1):32–41.
7. Miller DT, Adam MP, Aradhya S et al. Consensus statement: Chromosomal microarray is a first-tier clinical diagnostic test for individuals with developmental disabilities or congenital anomalies. *Am J Hum Genet.* 2010;86(5):749–64.
8. Newton CR, Graham A, Heptinstall LE et al. Analysis of any point mutation in DNA. The amplification refractory mutation system (ARMS). *Nucleic Acids Res.* 1989; 17(7):2503–16.
9. Liu X, Han S, Wang Z, Gelernter J, Yang BZ. Variant callers for next-generation sequencing data: A comparison study. *PLOS ONE.* 2013;8(9):e75619.
10. Bennett RL. The family medical history as a tool in preconception consultation. *J Community Genet.* 2012;3(3):175–83.
11. Allyse M, Minear MA, Berson E et al. Noninvasive prenatal testing: A review of international implementation and challenges. *Int J Womens Health.* 2015;7:113.
12. Elce A, Boccia A, Cardillo G et al. Three novel CFTR polymorphic repeats improve segregation analysis for cystic fibrosis. *Clin Chem.* 2009;55(7):1372–9.

13. Cariati F, Savarese M, D'Argenio V, Salvatore F, Tomaiuolo R. The SEeMORE strategy: Single-tube electrophoresis analysis-based genotyping to detect monogenic diseases rapidly and effectively from conception until birth. *Clin Chem Lab Med.* 2017;56(1):40–50.

14. Treff NR, Fedick A, Tao X, Devkota B, Taylor D, Scott Jr RT. Evaluation of targeted next-generation sequencing–based preimplantation genetic diagnosis of monogenic disease. *Fertil Steril.* 2013;99(5):1377–84.

15. Peters BA, Kermani BG, Alferov O et al. Detection and phasing of single base *de novo* mutations in biopsies from human *in vitro* fertilized embryos by advanced whole-genome sequencing. *Genome Res.* 2015;25(3):426–34.

16. Kung A, Munné S, Bankowski B, Coates A, Wells D. Validation of next-generation sequencing for comprehensive chromosome screening of embryos. *Reprod Biomed Online.* 2015;31(6):760–9.

Index

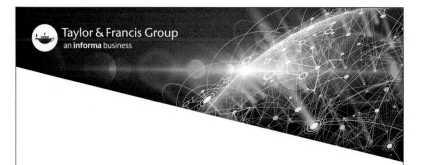